Human Response to Disaster: Health Promotion and Healing Following Catastrophic Events

Guest Editor

DANA BJARNASON, PhD, RN

CRITICAL CARE NURSING CLINICS OF NORTH AMERICA

www.ccnursing.theclinics.com

Consulting Editor
JANET FOSTER, PhD, RN, CNS

December 2010 • Volume 22 • Number 4

SAUNDERS an imprint of ELSEVIER, Inc.

W.B. SAUNDERS COMPANY
A Division of Elsevier Inc.

Elsevier Inc., 1600 John F. Kennedy Blvd., Suite 1800, Philadelphia, PA 19103-2899

http://www.theclinics.com

CRITICAL CARE NURSING CLINICS OF NORTH AMERICA Volume 22, Number 4
December 2010 ISSN 0899-5885, ISBN-13: 978-1-4557-0382-1

Editor: Katie Hartner
Developmental Editor: Donald Mumford

Critical Care Nursing Clinics of North America (ISSN 0899-5885) is published quarterly by Elsevier Inc., 360 Park Avenue South, New York, NY 10010-1710. Months of issue are March, June, September, and December. Business and Editorial Offices: 1600 John F. Kennedy Blvd., Suite 1800, Philadelphia, PA 19103-2899. Periodicals postage paid at New York, NY and additional mailing offices. Subscription prices are $135.00 per year for US individuals, $282.00 per year for US institutions, $71.00 per year for US students and residents, $180.00 per year for Canadian individuals, $353.00 per year for Canadian institutions, $206.00 per year for international individuals, $353.00 per year for international institutions and $104.00 per year for Canadian and foreign students/residents. To receive student/resident rate, orders must be accompanied by name of affiliated institution, data of term, and the *signature* of program/residency coordinator on institution letterhead. Orders will be billed at individual rate until proof of status is received. Foreign air speed delivery is included in all *Clinics* subscription prices. All prices are subject to change without notice. **POSTMASTER:** Send address changes to *Critical Care Nursing Clinics of North America*, Elsevier Health Sciences Division, Subscription Customer Service, 3251 Riverport Lane, Maryland Heights, MO 63043. **Customer Service: 1-800-654-2452 (US and Canada); 314-447-8871 (outside US and Canada). Fax: 314-447-8029. E-mail: JournalsCustomerService-usa@elsevier.com (for print support) and Journals OnlineSupport-usa@elsevier.com (for online support).**

Reprints. For copies of 100 or more of articles in this publication, please contact the Commercial Reprints Department, Elsevier Inc., 360 Park Avenue South, New York, New York, 10010-1710; Tel.: (212) 633-3813, Fax: (212) 462-1935, and E-mail: reprints@elsevier.com.

Critical Care Nursing Clinics of North America is covered in *MEDLINE/PubMed (Index Medicus), International Nursing Index, Nursing Citation Index, Cumulative Index to Nursing and Allied Health Literature, and RNdex Top 100.*

Printed in the United States of America
Transferred to Digital Printing, 2011

Contributors

CONSULTING EDITOR

JANET FOSTER, PhD, RN, CNS
Texas Woman's University, College of Nursing, Houston, Texas

GUEST EDITOR

DANA BJARNASON, PhD, RN
Associate Administrator & Chief Nursing Officer, Ben Taub General Hospital, Quentin Mease Community Hospital, Houston, Texas

AUTHORS

ELIZABETH CLOYD, MBA, RN, NEA-BC, FACHE
Executive Vice President/Chief Nurse Executive, Harris County Hospital District, Houston, Texas

CARMEL B. DYER, MD, FACP, AGSF
Roy M. and Phyllis Gough Huffington Chair in Gerontology, Professor and Executive Vice-Chairman of Internal Medicine, Director of the Division of Geriatric and Palliative Medicine, Executive Director of the Consortium on Aging, Chief, Geriatric and Palliative Medicine, Lyndon Baines Johnson General Hospital, University of Texas Medical School, Houston, Texas

MINI M. JOSE, PhD, RN
Assistant Professor, School of Nursing, University of Texas Medical Branch, Galveston, Texas

FRANCES KELLY, MSN, RN
Ben Taub General Hospital, Harris County Hospital District, Houston, Texas

ANNE S. LIONG, PhD, MBA, RN
Director, Nursing Standards and Policies, Nursing Practice and Professional Advancement, Harris County Hospital District, Houston, Texas

SAMUEL U. LIONG, MS, MBA, RN, PMP
Project Manager, School of Biomedical Informatics, University of Texas Health Science Center at Houston, Houston, Texas

THOMAS B. MENDEZ, PhD(c), MSN, RN, CNS
Assistant Professor, Baccalaureate Program, School of Nursing, University of Texas Medical Branch, Galveston, Texas

KAREN S. MIGL, PhD, RNC, WHNP-BC
Assistant Professor, Coordinator, RN-BSN Online Track, Richard and Lucille DeWitt School of Nursing, Stephen F. Austin State University, Nacogdoches, Texas

MICHAEL L. MISTRIC, PhD, RN, FNP, BC
Family Nurse Practitioner, Extended Care Line, Michael E. DeBakey Veterans Affairs
Medical Center; Adjunct Assistant Professor, Texas Woman's University, Houston, Texas

JOHN S. MURRAY, PhD, RN
Children's Hospital Boston, Boston, Massachusetts

ROSE M. POWELL, PhD, RN
Assistant Professor, Course Coordinator, Leadership in Nursing Systems, Richard and
Lucille DeWitt School of Nursing, Stephen F. Austin State University, Nacogdoches,
Texas

TOBIN A. SPARLING, JD
Professor of Law, South Texas College of Law, Houston, Texas

PAULA A. STANGELAND, BSN, RN, CRRN, PhDc
Clinical Instructor, University of Texas Medical Branch, School of Nursing, Galveston,
Texas

SHAINY B. VARGHESE, PhD, RN, CPNP
Assistant Professor of Nursing, University of Houston-Victoria, Sugar Land, Texas

Contents

> This article presents a review of the literature related to disaster prepared-
> ness and nursing. A definition of disaster as set forth by the American Red
> Cross is provided. Eight themes, including (1) defining disaster, (2) nursing
> during and after disaster, (3) nursing education in disaster preparedness,
> (4) military nurse preparedness, (5) postdisaster stress, (6) ethical issues
> and intent to respond, (7) policy, and (8) hospital emergency policy, were
> derived from the review and are explored in this article. Although a plethora
> of disaster-related literature exists, the voice of the nurses who worked
> during these disasters is missing. Areas of proposed research illuminated
> by current research are suggested.

> Emergency response providers–these groups are responsible for the pro-
> tection and preservation of life, property, evidence, as well as the environ-
> ment in the early stages of an incident. Emergency response providers
> need to be afforded with commensurate compensation, benefits, incen-
> tives, and protection to safeguard their welfare as well as assure support
> to their dependents and survivors if an injury, a permanent disability, or
> even death occurs. Such provisions encourage emergency response pro-
> vider participation and promotion of recruitment efforts that help to build
> and sustain more resilient emergency response provider communities
> throughout the country.

> Disasters arrive unexpectedly and in most cases, without warning. There
> are many physical and environmental issues that health care providers
> as first responders must consider when dealing with disasters. This article
> examines the physical and environmental issues that health care profes-
> sionals in the role of first responders may encounter during disasters or ex-
> treme emergencies. It is hoped that discussing this issue will help health
> care professionals to gain an understanding of the physical and environ-
> mental considerations during disasters and therefore to provide the care
> needed for healing and recovery for both their patients and themselves.

> Health care providers responding to the call of duty during catastrophic
> events are expected to provide culturally, ethically, and spiritually

competent care to disaster victims. Health care providers have many resources available to guide decision making and the provision of care during disasters. Familiarization with these resources is essential to the
provision of efficient and effective care under chaotic conditions. Health
care providers function in many roles, and the integration of local efforts
with teams of professionals who have specialized disaster response training from international agencies is the most appropriate approach to providing ethically sound, spiritually sensitive, and culturally appropriate
care to disaster victims. Disaster response interventions should be guided
by ethnocultural beliefs, and local networks should be consulted to manage ethnic sentiments. Ethical decision making should be based on sound
principles, and ethical dilemmas should be identified and resolved through
appropriate processes. Human beings are spiritual beings and everything
possible should be done to ease spiritual suffering during a disaster.

From 1900 there have been more than 9800 natural disasters affecting
more than 67 million children worldwide. Because of unique physical, developmental, and psychosocial characteristics of children, caring for them
during complex emergencies is different to caring for adults. However,
planning for these unique physical, developmental, and psychosocial
needs has not been well addressed when planning for complex emergencies. Therefore, the purpose of this article is to review those characteristics
of children that place them at higher disaster risk, and discuss the preparations necessary to meet their needs before, during, and in the aftermath
of complex emergencies.

Every time a disaster occurs, health care professionals question their preparation to meet the special needs of the most vulnerable casualties, children. This article identifies approaches that health care professionals
can use when caring for children and families in disasters, which best respond to their psychosocial needs.

Analysis of world disasters has provided valuable information on the psychological effect on those experiencing the disaster. However, little is
known about the response by those with established psychiatric or mental
health issues. This article explores the issues regarding disaster planning
and intervention for survivors with established psychiatric or mental health
issues.

Inhabitants of every region in the world are susceptible to natural disasters,
and for the last several years, the havoc wreaked by hurricanes, tsunamis,

and earthquakes on humans has dominated the news. This article presents the special needs of older adults in disaster situations to help nurses meet the challenges associated with serving this vulnerable population.

A disaster is defined as an unforeseen event that causes great damage, destruction, and human suffering, which in turn overwhelms the response capacity of local communities, oftentimes necessitating external requests for assistance on a national or international level. Many investigators have explored the nature of, reasons for, and management of disasters; however, there exists a paucity of literature that details disaster from the victims' perspective. This article focuses on the cultural, ethical, and spiritual implications of natural disasters from the survivors' perspective.

The experiences and lessons of catastrophic natural events in the 1980s and 1990s, including hurricanes, tornados, and earthquakes, as well as human-made events such as the terrorist attacks of 9/11 led to a focus on the "before-and-after" periods of disaster from the perspective of both the victim and the responder. Numerous books and articles describe the phases of disaster management in generalized terms and largely from the victim's perspective. In contrast, this article describes the 4 phases of disaster management, including (1) mitigation, (2) preparedness, (3) response, and (4) recovery from the perspective of a health care provider.

THE CLINICS ARE NOW AVAILABLE ONLINE!
Access your subscription at:
www.theclinics.com

Preface

Human Response: Health Promotion and Healing Before, During, and After Catastrophic Events

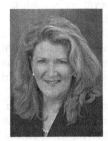

Dana Bjarnason, PhD, RN
Guest Editor

Fossilized evidence bears witness to the fact that since the beginning of time humankind has had to deal with the aftermath of catastrophic events. Over our lifetime, we learned about the cataclysmic events that shaped the very world we now inhabit, including volcanic activity and huge meteorites that changed life upon the earth. Studying the city of Pompeii, we were fascinated by the archaeological evidence that reveals the complete devastation of an entire city following the eruption of Mount Vesuvius, which happened so quickly that citizens, overwhelmed by the eruption, were captured forever, enveloped by volcanic ash. We ponder about the kind of event that wiped out the Mayan civilization of Central America. We read about the great plague, and these stories bring trepidation when in our time, the unexpected and deadly virus SARS or the threat of H1N1 flu disrupts travel, commerce, and healthcare around the world, and where—in addition to killing world citizens—it has devastating effects for healthcare providers caring for them.

In more recent times we have had to deal with the physical, mental, and emotional anguish of trauma brought on not by nature, but by humankind. The name Chernobyl—almost 25 years after the first major nuclear power plant disaster—is still familiar and the lasting effects of the explosion remain a problem for the health and welfare of an entire region and the people who live there.

Most people remember Oklahoma City where just fifteen years ago our sense of reality was turned upside down by a horrifying terroristic attack that left 169 people dead, 19 of them under the age of six. Many lessons were learned from health care

Crit Care Nurs Clin N Am 22 (2010) ix–xiii
doi:10.1016/j.ccell.2010.10.004
0899-5885/10/$ — see front matter © 2010 Elsevier Inc. All rights reserved.

providers attending to the dead and wounded then—but unfortunately, these lessons were not much use when, 6 years later, the next major terrorist attack to strike the United States did so with chilling premeditation and deadly accuracy. On September 11, 2001, we recall the scenes of health care providers standing at the ready, waiting to receive victims from the World Trade Center. Unfortunately the true suffering was to begin when the raw emotional reality set in—there were few survivors of the initial traumatic event—and it was a wounded city, a devastated country, and a stunned world that needed ministration.

Within the realm of natural disasters, it is not hard for any of us to recall the images from several recent large-scale tragedies that have shattered our sensibilities—from the Indonesian Tsunami—whose real death toll will probably never be known, but that is now reported to have taken over 230,000 lives—to Hurricane Ike, whose wrath changed the lives for millions of people living on the Gulf of Mexico. Even more recently, the earthquake in Haiti proved stirring as a global outpouring of relief sought to alleviate a decimated country's pain and suffering, and now, more recently still, the floods in Pakistan, which overwhelmed a country and have revealed to the world a very real and pressing concern in the form of donor fatigue.

The compelling story that prompts worldwide responses to catastrophic, headline-capturing events are laudable; however, the challenge lies in being able to facilitate the appropriate and prudent use of resources, as well as to ensure that the same supply, monetary, and humanitarian aid reaches those who are victims of situations that may not be as dramatic. A report published in 2004 provides data that show that nearly 1.5 million people died in earthquakes, volcanic eruptions, tropical storms, droughts, and other natural disasters between 1980 and 2000.[1] It is estimated that 184 people die per day from some form of disaster—numbers that do not draw the same kind of compelling support from the worldwide community. Major disasters pose serious threats to the fundraising capabilities of agencies that provide local relief to smaller, localized disasters. Testimony to this was the funding drain placed on many organizations (including larger organizations with global responsibilities) following the outpouring of support for World Trade Center victims. These unfortunate outcomes are chilling in view of the fact that there is a clear link between poverty and vulnerability in the face of disasters. In fact, the real killer is poverty, not the forces of nature. Although only 11% of people exposed to natural disasters live in poor countries, they account for more than 53% of the deaths.[1] Our goal as health care professionals must be to help these agencies use resources wisely by providing theory-driven, evidence-based research tools to fuel wise aid responses.

The impact of post-traumatic stress syndrome on the local, national, and worldwide community is ever more affected by globalization and the ability to visualize almost immediately the disturbing events associated with human suffering during and after catastrophes. Events that happen hundreds and thousands of miles away may have a severe impact on the health of people around the world. Evidence suggests that children in the United States who are suffering from post-traumatic stress disorder are among the least understood, under-studied, and inconsistently served groups.[2] The ramifications of this phenomenon as a worldwide dilemma are staggering.

In addition to concerns about the failure to identify and respond to the needs of children is the documented exploitation of vulnerable populations that runs rampant in the chaos and confusion that follows a disaster. Although most religious charities do not attach conditions to their aid—and many of the larger ones actually have policies against proselytizing—some smaller religious groups saw the event in Indonesia as an opportunity to plant Christian principles in 300 Muslim children who lost their parents in the tsunami. Similar concerns arose in Haiti, when both well-meaning and unscrupulous activities that served to separate children from there families were identified. The far-reaching effects of these types of endeavors relative to the loss of meaningful spiritual, cultural, and social connections may not be understood for years, if ever.

Another morbid issue that has received increasing attention is the matter of human trafficking. More than 140 years ago a devastating war was fought to rid our country of slavery; however, human slavery has returned as a growing global threat to the lives and freedom of millions of men, women, and children. Adults and children in forced labor, bonded labor, and commercial sexual servitude are estimated at 12.3 million people. There is substantial evidence that no country is immune from human trafficking and that 600,000–800,000 men, women, and children are trafficked across international borders each year. This figure does not include people trafficked within countries. Victims are forced into prostitution, or to work in quarries and sweatshops, on farms, as domestics, as child soldiers, and in many forms of involuntary servitude. Alarmingly, US Government estimates show that over half of all victims of international trafficking are trafficked for sexual exploitation.[3]

One of the seven reported drivers of human trafficking is a natural disaster. Given the propensity for a natural disaster to also be a harbinger of criminal elements, economic hardship, corrupt governments, social disruption, and political instability, five more forces increase the probability that human trafficking will be an issue associated with a disaster. Making this an even more compelling issue is the overwhelming United Nations estimate that places 21st century slave trade profits among the top three revenue sources for organized crime after trafficking in narcotics and arms.[4]

Evidence suggests that disaster losses, rather than stemming from unexpected events, are predictable results of three major systems: (a) the physical environment; (b) the social and demographic characteristics of the communities that experience them; and (c) the buildings, roads, bridges, and other components of the constructed environment.[5] Although the talents of nurses may not be able to greatly impact the physical environment or the infrastructure, our capabilities relative to understanding and impacting the human needs of communities is unprecedented. Indeed, Florence Nightingale led the way in the Crimea. Her nursing theories about the importance of hygiene, nutrition, autonomous nursing practice, frameworks for nursing preparation, and standards for ethical conduct and character have withstood the test of time and have been joined by other nursing and social science theories, research, and evidence-based practices that will enable us to continue to develop assessment and intervention strategies that positively impact humankind at its most desperate moments.

In 2005, I was pursuing doctoral studies at the University of Texas Medical Branch in Galveston, Texas. I was enrolled in GNRS 6345, the Study of Nursing Science, whose course description stated that:

This course emphasizes existing and evolving research focused on health promotion, human response, and healing. The analysis, critical evaluation, and interpretation of research in these areas provide students with the foundation to explore original ideas for the purpose of generating nursing knowledge. Research exemplars will be presented and discussed. Students will delineate areas of research consistent with the course focus. Evaluation is based on term papers, class presentations, and class participation.

My classmates and I were pondering an approach that would be interesting and innovative, while at the same time meeting the goal of generating nursing knowledge. Our minds were largely on the recent cataclysmic death and destruction that had occurred on December 26, 2004, when an undersea earthquake produced the horrifying tsunami that killed over 230,000 people in 14 countries, becoming one of the deadliest natural disasters to strike humankind in recorded history.[6] It seemed only natural that health care professionals living on a barrier island in the Gulf of Mexico would be interested in delving into the issue of human responses to catastrophic events. As we discussed and debated, our thoughts began to coalesce around the idea of a 4-hour seminar which we eventually entitled "A Disaster Dialogue: A Symposium Exploring Human Responses Experienced by Victims and Healthcare Providers Following Catastrophic Events." We posed to ourselves the following questions:

- How do we help the victims of catastrophic events and health care providers who provide care for them deal with the ramifications of the event: the shattered bodies, the ravaged minds, and the raw emotions?
- How do we prepare ourselves to deal with people—angry because their mother, the sea, who has given them life by providing their livelihoods, has just wiped out entire communities and, even more soberly, an entire generation?
- How do we prepare ourselves to deal with our own unreality—witnessing and participating in nightmarish circumstances that include not only traumatic injuries and emotional strife, but the daily problem of finding fresh food and clean water?
- How can we use these experiences to employ and build upon the scientific body of work that has begun to address the best theory-driven research and evidence-based health promotion, healing, and human responses to catastrophic events?

Little did we know the prescience of our actions—within 8 months of our discussions, our lives would be significantly affected by Hurricane Katrina—which would make landfall on August 29, 2005 and be recognized as one of the deadliest and costliest hurricanes ever to occur.[7] As I watched the drama unfold in this and subsequent natural and human-made disasters, I realized that the symposium we had developed and presented addressed the significant issues that affect human populations following catastrophic events. Then, in 2008, the work we did became a lived experience as Hurricane Ike damaged and destroyed much of the city of Galveston, a place I call home. Despite the resilient circumstances of my life, the impact on me was overwhelming, and I believed that publishing our work for other nurses was an important next step; therefore, I was thrilled when I was given the opportunity to edit a journal focused specifically on human response to disasters. I appreciate that many of my fellow classmates were eager to join me in turning their oral presentations into a written manuscript. I also am indebted to others who agreed to cover topics that could not be overlooked, including the very real and special needs of the elderly, the young, and those with mental illnesses.

As health care professionals, as nurse clinicians, and as nurse scholars—it is imperative that we build on existing theories and develop new theories to advance the science of nursing. We need not look far to begin—take, for example, Bandura's Self-Efficacy Theory, which has shown potential for wide application in learning and development situations. It takes full account of external physical and social structures as well as internal cognitive processes. It is a theory which is simultaneously realistic and humanistic. Or, take Fishbein's Theory of Reasoned Action, which provides a framework for identifying key behavioral and normative beliefs affecting behavior and has been used successfully to predict and explain a wide variety of health behaviors and intentions such as smoking, drinking, exercise, seat belt use, safety helmet use, and breastfeeding—does it have a useful application in disaster planning? Perhaps we will turn to the Conservation of Resources Theory—a theory that is used to predict the consequences of positive and negative changes. The need to explore the use of Leininger's Theory of Transcultural Care is implied by the very nature of an adequate response to global disaster relief. Last but not least, we rely on nursing theory derived from the mother of nursing—Florence Nightingale, whose work continues to have real implications for disaster management.

Although the fate of those who lost their lives is clear, the impact of disasters on survivors is less so. The articles in this journal bring to you a dialogue that examines the scope of catastrophic events, examining the very real impact on the victims of disasters and health care providers who respond to the call of duty. We examine and offer evidence-based research and the lived experience about what works and what does not. It is important work, for it somehow seems imperative that those of us with the "know how" should know "how to."

I would like to acknowledge those individuals who made this journal possible by thanking Alice Hill, PhD, RN, Professor, University of Texas Medical Branch Graduate School of Biomedical Sciences Nursing Doctoral Program, and the Class of GNRS 6345, Spring 2005: Leah Best, Pat Brenza, Shainy Varghese, Margaret Ottenbacher, Jennifer Kelly, Rosie Morales, Mary Gordon, Mini Jose, Anne Liong, Karen Migl, Karen O'Brien, Michael Mistric, and Thom Mendez for their contribution to the 2005 symposium.

Dana Bjarnason, PhD, RN
Ben Taub General Hospital
Quentin Mease Community Hospital
1504 Taub Loop
Houston, TX 77030, USA

E-mail address:
dana_bjarnason@hchd.tmc.edu

REFERENCES

1. United Nations Development Program. Reducing disaster risk: A challenge for development. Available at: http://www.undp.org/cpr/disred/documents/publications/rdr/english/rdr_english.pdf. Accessed October 6, 2010.
2. Perry BD. Traumatized children: How childhood trauma influences brain development. J Calif Alliance Ment Ill 2000;11(1):48–51.
3. U.S. Department of Health and Human Services. Human trafficking into and within the United States: A review of the literature. Available at: http://aspe.hhs.gov/hsp/07/HumanTrafficking/LitRev/index.pdf. Accessed October 6, 2010.
4. U.S. Department of State. Trafficking in persons report. Available at: http://www.state.gov/documents/organization/34158.pdf. Accessed October 6, 2010.
5. Mileti DS. Disasters by design: A reassessment of natural hazards in the United States. Washington, DC: Joseph Henry Press; 1999.
6. Guy Carpenter & Company. Tsunami: Indian Ocean event and investigation into potential global risks. Available at: http://www.guycarp.com/portal/extranet/pdf/Tsunami_Report_Final.pdf. Accessed October 6, 2010.
7. U.S. Department of Commerce. Hurricane Katrina. Most destructive hurricane every to strike the U.S. Available at: http://www.katrina.noaa.gov/. Accessed October 6, 2010.

Disaster Nursing: A Retrospective Review

Paula A. Stangeland, BSN, RN, CRRN, PhDc

KEYWORDS

• Nursing • Disaster • Hurricane • Posttraumatic stress
• Preparedness

Natural disasters are destructive forces of nature that severely affect human lives as well as the environment. Catastrophic health emergencies including human-made and natural disasters usually result in mass casualties that require hospitals to increase capacity.[1,2] However, to increase capacity and provide quality patient care, facilities must have adequate staffing. Researchers have shown that health care professionals (HCP), including nurses, physicians, and dentists, feel responsible for responding to disasters; however, these same studies indicate that approximately 40% of health care professionals reported that they would not respond during health emergencies.[3,4]

Nurses' intent to respond to disasters is a topic that has not been exhaustively researched. It is prudent to understand nurses' intent to respond, as the capacity of hospitals is directly related to the number of staff nurses available to care for the influx of patients during disasters.[5] Because nurses are invaluable to disaster response efforts, more research is necessary to validate findings of recent studies and clarify the needs of nurses who respond to disasters and other health emergencies. Existing literature does not adequately describe the needs of nurses while working during disaster situations, nor is it clear why nurses do or do not respond. Further complicating nursing's response to emergencies is the influence of the nursing shortage and the identified lack of education preparing nurses for disaster response, making these recommended areas for further exploration.[6]

REVIEW OF THE LITERATURE

The purpose of this article is to provide a critique of published works that are representative of research studies that have explored disaster preparedness related to nursing. In addition, rationale for conducting future research in the area of nurses' experiences of intent to respond and working during major disasters is discussed. An extensive review of the literature was completed using health care literature databases including

The author has nothing to disclose.
University of Texas Medical Branch, School of Nursing, 301 University Boulevard, Galveston, TX 77555-1029, USA
E-mail address: pastange@utmb.edu

Crit Care Nurs Clin N Am 22 (2010) 421–436
doi:10.1016/j.ccell.2010.09.003
0899-5885/10/$ – see front matter © 2010 Elsevier Inc. All rights reserved.

CINAHL, Medline (Ovid), PubMed, and PsycINFO. In 1974, the Robert T. Stafford Disaster Relief Act was signed into law, establishing the process by which presidents could declare disasters in states overwhelmed by catastrophic events. Therefore, the literature review was limited to the past 36 years. Keywords entered into the databases were nursing, disaster, hurricane, posttraumatic stress, and preparedness. The search revealed a vast amount of disaster-related literature, which was categorized into 8 thematic sections: (a) defining disaster, (b) nursing during and after disaster, (c) nursing education in disaster preparedness, (d) military nurse preparedness, (e) postdisaster stress, (f) ethical issues and intent to respond, (g) policy, and (h) hospital emergency policy.

DEFINING DISASTER

The association between disasters and human existence is indisputable, hence many definitions for disaster are found in the literature. A comprehensive definition for disaster is difficult to locate in the literature—most definitions are either too broad or too narrow, and many organizations have created their own definitions for the term. For the purpose of this review, the definition of the term that was deemed most appropriate was that used by the American Red Cross (ARC), which defines disaster as:

> A threatening or occurring event of such destructive magnitude and force as to dislocate people, separate family members, damage or destroy homes, and injure or kill people. A disaster produces a range and level of immediate suffering and basic human needs that cannot be promptly or adequately addressed by the affected people, and impedes them from initiating and proceeding with their recovery efforts. Natural disasters include floods, tornadoes, hurricanes, typhoons, winter storms, tsunamis, hail storms, wildfires, windstorms, epidemics, and earthquakes. Human-caused disasters—whether intentional or unintentional—include residential fires, building collapses, transportation accidents, hazardous materials releases, explosions, and domestic acts of terrorism.[7]

Common to all definitions of disaster is the characteristic that disasters are destructive events that more often than not require assistance from outside the community.

NURSING DURING AND AFTER DISASTER

Researchers report that nurses are one of the largest groups of emergency responders during a disaster and are at risk for psychosocial problems that may need interventions to help them cope with exposure to disasters.[8,9] In the immediate aftermath of a disaster, the effects can be overwhelming to nurses working in the area, as there is a great deal of chaos and confusion that nurses must contend with and overcome.[8,10–12]

Studies indicate disaster emergencies create an atmosphere of pandemonium and uncertainty and that nurses perceive they have been or will be abandoned by leadership.[8,10,12,13] Feelings of abandonment by management and a lack of communication play a major role in the decision-making processes of nurses and other HCPs when deciding to work during a disaster.[13–15] Nurses state that they feel disaster plans are made by leaders or managers without input from the nurses who will actually be working and taking care of patients during and after the disaster.[8,12]

Giarratano and colleagues[8] conducted an interpretive phenomenological study based on van Manen's "lived experience" philosophy. The sample included 16 perinatal nurses who worked during Hurricane Katrina. The purpose of the study was to make explicit the perinatal nurses' shared meanings of their lived experience of providing care in New Orleans during Hurricane Katrina. Major themes that emerged from the study include (a) duty to care, (b) conflicts in duty, (c) uncertain times, (d) strength to endure, (e) grief, (f) anger, and (g) feeling right again. Findings demonstrated that nurses who work during disasters must live through the uncertainty of the situation and be prepared to adapt to the needs that arise in both patient care and self-preservation situations. This study revealed that primary resources needed by nurses while working during a disaster include excellent basic nursing skills, intuitive problem solving, and a sense of staff unity. Researchers noted that the nurses exhibited a wide range of problems related to stress. These problems included changed sleep patterns, change in mood, eating problems, substance abuse, and avoidance behaviors. At the same time, it was recognized that the nurse participants practiced in harmony with duty to care values and demonstrated behaviors of strength, courage, and resilience.[8]

O'Boyle and colleagues[13] completed a qualitative study with a purposive sample of 33 nurses who participated in focus groups ranging from 2 to 9 participants in each group. The sample of nurses was recruited from 3 Midwest hospitals that were designated as receiving sites for evacuees. The purpose of the study was to identify beliefs and concerns of nurses who worked in hospitals designated as receiving sites during public health emergencies. Abandonment was the major theme that emerged from the focus group interviews. This theme was supported by subthemes including: chaos, unsafe environment, loss of freedom, and limited institutional commitment. Nurses felt that policies were not well thought out, and that they were left out of the communication loop. In addition, the nurses stated that they did not receive any preparedness training to handle bioterrorist events.[13] Nurses believed that in the event of a bioterrorist attack, there would be a disruption in normal staffing resources. Aware that nurse staffing under normal conditions is at times already strained, the nurses feared that they would not be free to leave the workplace. Therefore, these researchers reported that the participants in the study believed that a shortage of nursing staff would be indirectly related to nurses who refused to work during a disaster. A limitation of this study is the small number of participants in some of the focus groups, which might have limited the discussions.

A qualitative descriptive study completed by Broussard and colleagues[10] explored school nurses' feelings and experiences working in the aftermath of Hurricanes Katrina and Rita. The sample consisted of 41 female school nurses from across the state of Louisiana who attended an Annual School Nurse Conference held in March 2006. Nurse participants had an average age 48 years. Researchers reported that the participants were from all areas of Louisiana, including areas that were not in the path of either hurricane. Participants were asked one question: "Please share your experiences and feelings about Hurricanes Katrina and/or Rita".[10] In addition to the qualitative question, demographic data were collected that included: (a) age, (b) years of experience as a school nurse, (c) gender, (d) support systems loss or damage to home and vehicle, (e) damage to school, and (f) change in work assignment as a result of the storm. Data analysis was not described; however, findings were categorized into 2 major themes: personal impact and professional impact. Personal impact included 3 subthemes: (a) uncertainty, (b) helplessness, and (c) thankfulness. Professional impact included 2 themes: practice challenges and practice rewards. The participants portrayed a wide array of emotions and feelings that were similar to previous studies. Researchers recommended that all school nurses would benefit from having both formal and informal support systems and mental health services available to them in the aftermath of future hurricanes.[10] Identifying the philosophic underpinnings as well as the method for data analysis and rigor would have strengthened the validity of this study.

NURSING EDUCATION IN DISASTER PREPAREDNESS

Although some nurses identified their experiences of working during and in the aftermath of Hurricane Katrina and other health emergencies as rewarding, they also identified planning and education as critical needs for providing care in future disasters.[3,9–11] Hughes and colleagues[9] report that nurses believe that they need to be involved at the onset of the emergency planning process. During emergencies, nurses stated that they used their most basic skills and teamwork when providing patient care, but recognized that further education is necessary to enhance their knowledge prior to future events.[3,8,11]

According to the International Nursing Coalition for Mass Casualty Education (INCMCE), every nurse must have sufficient knowledge and skill to recognize the potential for a mass casualty incident.[16] In addition, the INCMCE states that every nurse must be able to identify when a mass casualty event may have occurred, know how to protect oneself, know how to provide immediate care for those individuals involved, and be able to recognize their own role and limitations during such a disaster. The INCMCE also recommends that nurses know where to seek additional educational information and how to access resources.[16]

The position of the American Nurses Association (ANA) related to practice during disaster is that all nurses are individually accountable for their actions and should practice according to their code of ethics.[17,18] Despite that the ANA acknowledges that working during disasters places nurses in unusual situations and conditions, the organization's code of ethics defines and directs the responsibilities of all practicing nurses regardless of the situation or setting. However, in the 2010 draft of the scope and standards of practice, the ANA recognizes that these standards may change during times of disaster.[19]

The Essentials of Baccalaureate Education for Professional Nursing Practice was created by The American Association of Colleges of Nursing (AACN).[20] This document provides guidelines for baccalaureate-level nursing schools to prepare students for disaster response. The AACN mandates that the baccalaureate nursing education curriculum contain emergency-preparedness and disaster-response information.[20] Specifically, the guidelines state that baccalaureate nursing programs should prepare graduates to use clinical judgment appropriately and provide timely interventions when making decisions and performing nursing care during disasters, mass casualties, and other emergency situations. In addition, nursing students should understand their role and participation in emergency preparedness and disaster response with an awareness of environmental factors and the risks these factors pose to self and patients.[20] It is not known whether the voices of nurses experienced in disaster have informed these essentials of education.

Educational competencies for associate degree nurses were created by the National League for Nurses (NLN) with support from the National Organization of Associate Degree Nursing.[21] Although the document provides core competencies that all associate degree nurses must meet, it does not specifically explicate the responsibilities of associate degree nurses during emergency situations. A particular skill indirectly related to disaster preparedness includes the ability to adapt patient care to changing health care environments.[21]

Gebbie and Qureshi,[22] well-known nurse experts in disaster management, maintain that it is necessary for all nurses to be prepared during disasters. These experts define the difference between emergency and disaster, and state that disasters disrupt many services and cause unforeseen threats to public health. These researchers further describe disasters as requiring assistance from outside the affected community. Gebbie and Qureshi,[22] at the request of the Centers for Disease Control and Prevention (CDC), developed 14 core emergency preparedness competencies for nurses. Although these competencies were developed by nurses; it is not known whether they have been incorporated or implemented in any educational program or facility where nurses work.

Research has shown that nursing schools may be lacking in the area of preparing students for disaster nursing.[23,24] Jennings-Saunders and colleagues[23] completed a descriptive survey study that investigated nursing students' perceptions regarding disaster nursing. One purpose of the study was to propose recommendations to help advance the discipline of nursing and nurse clinicians. A convenience sample of 51 senior nursing students participated. Each participant completed the Disaster Nursing Perception Questionnaire and the Demographic Profile Form. Data were analyzed for meaning and relationships of words using the data analysis technique of Morgan and Baxter. This study revealed that nursing students do not comprehend what disaster nursing means and why it is important to know what community resources are available during times of disaster. Furthermore, the study revealed that it is not known to what extent nursing faculties teach disaster preparedness in nursing programs, even though it is required.

Weiner and colleagues[24] administered an on-line survey to 2103 United States nursing program deans and nursing program directors to assess the level of disaster preparedness curricula in United States nursing schools. Only 348 surveys (17%) were completed and returned. This low response rate was identified as a limitation of the study. Baccalaureate and associate degree nursing programs made up more than 77% of the response rate. The study revealed that faculty was inadequately prepared to teach disaster preparedness and that most programs were overly saturated, leaving little room for disaster-preparedness education. A significant finding revealed that United States nursing school program curricula were limited in the area of disaster preparedness.

This review of the literature revealed that nursing school governing bodies have developed competencies to be included in the nursing curriculum; however, nursing programs have been identified as still lacking in the area of disaster nursing curriculum. In addition, studies reveal that nursing faculty members are not prepared to teach disaster nursing. Education of faculty in the area of disaster preparedness and response is an area that requires added consideration to adequately prepare students for disaster situations that may arise in the students' future careers.

MILITARY NURSE PREPAREDNESS

Military nursing has played a critical role in the history if nursing. Including data related to military nursing further enriches this review by addressing a significant area related to disaster and emergency preparation for nurses. Nurses' involvement in war-zone care dates back to the Crimean War in the 1800s, when Florence Nightingale cared for injured soldiers and introduced modern nursing during times of war. Researchers today posit that nursing during wartime has increased the profession's understanding of caring and responding during disasters.[24] It is recognized today that military nursing is challenged by working in diverse situations. Yet, according to recent studies, literature does not adequately describe military disaster nursing.[25]

On December 8, 1941, the United States declared war on Japan after the bombing of Pearl Harbor. Trapped in the midst of this war were 99 army and navy nurses who had no combat training. These nurses were caught in the middle of the battle on Bataan, a province of the Philippines. A few of the nurses escaped by boat but 77 were captured by the Japanese and held captive for 3 years in the Philippines. These nurses represent the first group of women in the military to be imprisoned by enemy forces.[26]

Elizabeth Norman[26] had the privilege of interviewing 20 of the 77 female nurses and wrote a book titled *We Band of Angels: The Untold Story of American Nurses Trapped on Bataan by the Japanese*. Norman began her study in 1990 and discovered that only 48 of the nurses were still living. During this study, she also found that most of the nurses had joined the military seeking adventure and romance. The nurses interviewed by Norman reported that the Philippine Islands were paradise until the war broke out and they were captured and held prisoner.

Norman[26] realized and reported that the nurses always started the conversation with humor but the interview soon found the nurses talking about the painful memories, with a few interviews ending in tears. During the study it was reported that all the nurses had similar accounts of the ordeal of being held captive and that all of the nurses answered the interview questions using "we" instead of "I." These comments led Norman to realize that the nurses viewed "unit cohesiveness" as their most important survival tool.[26]

Baker and colleagues,[27] using a self-report questionnaire, studied the stresses experienced by female nurses in Vietnam. A sample of 60 female Army nurses was recruited to complete this study. Findings revealed that 60% of the participating nurses reported they were poorly prepared by the military to serve in Vietnam. Also, registered nurses with less than 2 years of clinical experience before going to Vietnam were more likely to experience posttraumatic stress syndrome (PTSD) than nurses with more years of experience. The investigators identified the use of a self-report questionnaire as a study limitation, noting that the nurses had to recall events that occurred between 14 to 22 years prior to the study, adding to possible response bias. Baker and colleagues concluded that more research in this area is necessary.

Ravella[28] completed a descriptive study using a voluntary sample of 20 Air Force nurses in San Antonio, Texas, who served in Vietnam at various times during the Vietnam War. This study used in-depth interviews to gain insight into individual nurse perceptions of their wartime experiences, coping skills, and significant events that they remembered. Findings revealed that 25% of the participants described symptoms of PTSD. Participants also reported crucial survival skills including strong social support, maturity, nursing experience, humor, religion, and relaxation. The most significant events remembered were directly related to patient care situations and threats to survival. These events were reported by 60% of the nurses interviewed. Lastly, all of the nurses interviewed reported that their most rewarding professional experience was serving in the Vietnam War.[28]

Using a qualitative design, Stanton and colleagues[29] examined and compared experiences of nurses who served during World War II, the Korean War, the Vietnam War, and Operation Desert Storm. A sample of 22 nurses who volunteered to participate in the study were interviewed and asked to describe their experiences of serving during wartime. These researchers revealed that military nursing is an experience that is very different from community nursing. The 5 common themes that emerged from the study were: (a) reacting personally to the war experience, (b) living in the military, (c) the meaning of nursing in the military, (d) the social context of war, and (e) images and sensations of war.

In 2006 a proposed model for military disaster nursing was developed.[25] This model included actions deemed necessary during the 3 phases of disaster: (a) preparedness, (b) response, and (c) recovery. Military nurses possess a wide range of skills and are usually leaders in patient care. According to Wynd,[25] future disasters will encompass a wide range of disasters causing diverse mass casualties. Wynd also emphasized that more research is necessary to determine whether this proposed model for military disaster nursing will be useful during military as well as civilian disasters.

Although both can be stressful and traumatic, the literature reviewed revealed that nursing in the military is different from community disaster nursing. Because the literature reveals that working during disasters and traumatic situations causes increased stress for nurses, it is necessary to include information related to disorders that have been associated with experiencing traumatic situations.

POSTDISASTER STRESS

Working during disasters can have an immense impact on responders. It has been recognized in the literature that PTSD can develop soon after experiencing a traumatic event.[30] During times of disaster, caregivers and first responders react immediately to address physical injuries. However, these same caregivers have a tendency to react slowly or ignore injuries to themselves that are concealed deep within the consciousness. The National Institute of Mental Health (NIMH) defines PTSD as:

An anxiety disorder that can develop after exposure to a terrifying event or ordeal in which grave physical harm occurred or was threatened. Traumatic events that may trigger PTSD include violent personal assaults, natural or human-caused disasters, accidents, or military combat.[31]

According to the NIMH, PTSD can start at any time after experiencing a traumatic event. Symptoms of PTSD include bad dreams, flashbacks from the traumatic event, feeling like the traumatic incident is happening again, terrifying thoughts that one cannot control, staying away from places and things that are reminders of the event, feeling worried, guilty, or sad, feeling alone, problems sleeping, feeling on edge, angry outbursts, and thoughts of hurting oneself or others.[31,32]

Traumatic stress can change lives forever.[33] Researchers report that long-term dissociative and PTSD symptoms may occur after natural disasters.[34,35] In addition; survivors of disaster experience traumatic stress and the sights, sounds, and smells of the disaster are embedded in their minds forever.[33]

Acute stress disorder (ASD) is a condition that has a close relationship to PTSD. Researchers have documented that women are at higher risk for developing ASD and PTSD than men who have experienced traumatic events.[31,36] Laposa and colleagues[37] completed a secondary data analysis study addressing the correlation between sources of workplace stress and PTSD symptoms. The study sample included 51 emergency department employees located in urban Canada. Seventy-three percent of the participants were identified as nurses. PTSD was assessed using the Posttraumatic Stress Diagnostic Scale (PDS). Stress was measured using the Health Professionals' Stress Inventory—Revised (HPSI-R). Both scales were reported to have a Cronbach alpha of .80 or higher, which is adequate for internal consistency. Major findings included that 12% of the participants met all of the criteria for PTSD. Eighty-two percent of the respondents confirmed they did not attend debriefing sessions provided by the hospital and 100% of the respondents reported they did not receive professional help for stress outside of the workplace. In addition, results revealed that 20% of the participants reported they had considered changing jobs after stressful incidents. Researchers concluded that this study supports the need for employers to provide emotional support for workers who have experienced working during disaster or other traumatizing events that may lead to long-term emotional upset.[37]

Hughes and colleagues[9] completed a review of the literature to describe nursing's contribution to the psychosocial recovery of survivors of emergencies during all stages of disaster preparedness and recovery over a long-term period. The purpose of the integrative review was to provide guidance to nurses who are involved in emergency planning and response during the acute phase of an emergency. A second objective of the study was to inform nurses of the psychosocial effects that they may experience as health care providers working during disaster situations. These researchers revealed that nurses may experience stress-related psychosocial consequences that continue well past the disaster. Relevant factors that must be taken into account are: (a) level of exposure to the disaster, (b) environmental or working conditions and management practices, (c) nurses' perceptions and individual coping and stress reduction practices, and (d) the amount and type of training and previous experience. Hughes and colleagues[9] state that nurses are the largest entity of the emergency response team and need to be included from the beginning of emergency planning. Nurse responders must also undergo extensive education on the potential psychosocial symptoms that may be experienced as a result of working during a disaster.

When entire communities are affected by disaster, it is not possible to maintain previously normal daily activities. Conner and colleagues[30] suggest that identifying persons at risk for PTSD may improve outcomes after exposure to disasters and trauma. In addition, it is recognized that many screening and assessment instruments exist that measure PTSD after disaster; however, the validity of these instruments is unclear and more research is needed to verify their appropriateness. Brewin and colleagues[38] state that in order for PTSD screening instruments to be useful, they must be brief, consist of the minimum number of items necessary for accurate identification, and be written in a language that is easy to read. Furthermore, the symptoms of PTSD and ASD that may be experienced by nurses responding specifically to a major hurricane disaster may be different. Thus, one must first explore these perspectives by asking those who actually did respond and work in an affected facility. Only then will researchers begin to understand why nurses may elect not to respond during future hurricanes.

ETHICAL ISSUES AND INTENT TO RESPOND

Conflicting issues between family and self, safety, and work obligations often make it difficult for nurses and other HCPs to decide to work during a disaster.[12,39,40] Ethical opinions vary widely regarding decisions to report to duty during times of disaster and other health emergencies. The duty to report to work in health emergencies remains an intense topic of discussion in the health care arena. As unparalleled demands are placed on nurses and other HCPs who are called to work during disasters, some believe that the code of ethics for health care workers should specifically define the responsibilities of the HCP.[40] While the American Medical Association (AMA) and the Canadian Medical Association (CMA) have addressed the issue of responsibilities of physicians in their code of ethics, some researchers believe that it remains to be determined whether other health care professions will follow the same course of action in addressing the issue of providing care during health emergencies.[40]

The ANA revised the code of ethics for nurses to include interpretive statements to accommodate nurses' comprehensive role in the health care environment.[17] Because nurses are continually confronted with many challenges including unpredictable and complex medical and emergent conditions that affect both individuals and communities, the revised code of ethics addresses some of the more complex ethical obligations of nurses. The ANA code of ethics does not explicitly detail the obligation of nurses to report to duty during emergencies; however, it does address nurses' responsibilities to the public. One such responsibility outlined in the ANA code of ethics is that nurses have an obligation to "participate in institutional and legislative efforts to promote health and meet national health objectives."[17]

In an effort to examine ethical issues that arise during a pandemic disaster, Ehrenstein and colleagues[41] completed a quantitative survey design study. Surveys were sent to 1898 health care workers (HCWs) at a university hospital in Regensburg, Germany. Only 644 surveys were returned and of the 644 returned surveys, 264 of these HCWs were nurses. The purpose of the study was to solicit opinions of employees on professional ethics of proper response to pandemic influenza. Researchers discovered that 182 (28%) of the 644 HCWs surveyed believed that it was professionally acceptable to abandon the workplace to protect themselves and their family during a pandemic.[41] In addition, 77% of the respondents disagreed that HCWs should be permanently dismissed for not reporting to work during a pandemic, and 21% of the participants believed that HCWs without children should care primarily for the influenza patients. The researchers concluded that HCWs would benefit from further education regarding efficacy and availability of medications during a pandemic. It was also recognized that professional ethical guidelines are needed to help HCWs fulfill their duties in cases of pandemics.[41] Although this study revealed interesting information regarding the HCW's willingness to report to work during a pandemic, the survey used to complete the study was a newly developed instrument, and reliability and validity have not been established.

Qureshi and colleagues[39] completed a quantitative survey design study using a 23-item questionnaire. The sample consisted of 6428 HCP in the New York area. The purpose of this study was to assess the ability and willingness of HCPs in New York City to report to work during different types of catastrophic events. This study revealed that 47.9% of the participants reported the most frequent reason for employees' unwillingness to report to duty during a disaster was a fear and concern for the safety of their family and themselves. In addition, 82.5% of participants reported that they were most likely to report to duty in cases of mass casualty. However, 20% of the participants reported that they were not sure of their ability or willingness to report to duty during any catastrophic event. The researchers reported that a majority of the 6428 HCP participants in the New York area said they were least likely to report to duty in the case of severe acute respiratory syndrome (48.4%), radiation (57.3%), chemical terrorism (67.7%), and smallpox (61.1%). A reported limitation to this study is that it was conducted only in New York and cannot be generalized to other populations.[39]

Using a survey design, Balicer and colleagues[3] explored public health workers' perceptions toward working during an influenza pandemic as well as factors that may influence intent to respond if such an event occurred. The survey was sent to 531 employees of 3 major health departments in Maryland, with a return of 308 surveys. Clinical staff, nurses, physicians, and dentists accounted for 102 of the respondents. Data were analyzed using logistic regression to evaluate the association of demographic variables, and attitudes and beliefs with self-described likelihood of reporting to work during a pandemic disaster. The researchers studied the association between attitudes and beliefs related to pandemic preparedness and the self-reported likelihood of reporting to work. Of the 308 participants, only 163 (53.8%) stated that they would most likely report to work during a pandemic emergency. Forty percent noted that they would be asked by their health department to respond during an influenza pandemic event. Balicer and colleagues[3] reported that 66% of all participants perceived themselves to be at risk when performing their duties during a pandemic event. It was concluded that to reduce the perceived personal threat during a pandemic and increase the likelihood of employees responding during influenza pandemics, HCPs would benefit from continuing education regarding pandemics. These individuals must be assured that adequate protective equipment and psychological support would be made available to responders. Researchers also concluded that if employees are unwilling to respond during an influenza pandemic emergency, this behavior may cause a considerable deficit in national emergency response plans. Limitations to this study include the use of a subjective self-report survey and subject recruitment from 3 clinics in Maryland, therefore findings cannot be generalized to other populations. Lastly, the power of the study was not reported.[3]

Grimes and Mendias[42] completed a descriptive study that examined nurses' intentions to respond to an infectious disease emergency. This study was guided by Icek Ajzen's Theory of Planned Behavior. A sample of 313 licensed nurses in Texas who completed a state board of nursing mandated 2-hour bioterrorism continuing education class were recruited to participate in this study. Data were collected using 3 researcher-developed questionnaires. The Statistical Package for the Social Sciences (SPSS) version 16 was used to analyze data. According to the researchers, 292 participants completed all 3 questionnaires. The sample included both registered nurses (98%) and licensed vocational nurses (2%), with the majority being female (87%). Only 25% of the nurses who reported that they had a professional duty to respond also had a high intent-to-respond score. This significant finding raises concerns about adequate staffing during times of bioterrorism disasters or infectious disease events.

James and colleagues[43] completed a quantitative cross-sectional study with a sample of 291 nurses who worked during Hurricane Katrina in Mississippi. The purpose of this study was to evaluate the impact of Hurricane Katrina with respect to age on Mississippi nurses who worked during Hurricane Katrina. Nurses' ages in this sample ranged from 23 to 73 years. The sample was divided into 2 groups according to age: Group 1 was 23 to 45 years old and Group 2 was 46 to 73 years old. The researchers reported that there was a significant positive association between nurses aged 43 to 73 years and the development of poststorm depression, anxiety, PTSD, and lower health status when compared with nurses who were 23 to 45 years old. Older nurses developed more symptoms of stress-related disorders than the younger nurses. It was concluded that taking into consideration the growing shortage of nurses in the United States, it is important to understand how working during stressful situations affects older nurses, as retention of older nurses is important as a short-term resolution to the nursing shortage. This study used 7 self-report scales to gather data, which can be considered a limitation of the study. Self-report questionnaires are an excellent method to gain knowledge about a participant's feelings or beliefs; however, data gathered through self-report relies on the accuracy of the participant's subjective account and may also reveal socially desirable responses.[44] The findings of this study relied solely on self-reported data; hence, the results must be reviewed with caution.

Individuals as well as whole communities are greatly affected by any type of disaster emergency; whether it is natural or human-made.[9] A study performed by Brodie and colleagues[14] reported that there were approximately 21,700 Hurricane Katrina evacuees from New Orleans displaced to Houston, Texas. Following Hurricane Katrina, the CDC and the Louisiana Department of Health and Hospitals reported that there were 7543 nonfatal injuries such as cuts, broken bones, and animal bites secondary to clean-up efforts after Hurricane Katrina between September 8 and October 14, 2005.[45] These incidents make it clear that there is an unquestionable need for nurses to understand the importance of their response in times of disaster emergencies.

Conflicts of duty to family and work are further complicated by reports of nurses who have lost their jobs for not reporting to duty during times of emergency and impending disaster.[12,39,46] In addition to conflicts of duty to family and work, there is growing concern among HCPs that there is a lack of obligation in the duty of care during emergencies.[40]

DISASTER POLICY

Natural disasters cannot be prevented; however, damage caused by the event may be reduced if advanced action is taken to curtail risk and vulnerability to potentially affected communities. Government policies have attempted to address the issue of disaster relief and assistance to communities after large-scale disasters. To better understand disaster-related policy, it is important to review policies that directly impact society as a whole.

Disasters cause a disruption in government and community functions of affected areas. Because of this disruption of functions, Congress created and passed The Robert T. Stafford Disaster Relief and Emergency Relief Act. This public law authorizes the President of the United States to declare that a state of emergency or a major disaster exists. A stipulation to the president's authority is that the governor of the state(s) affected must request a declaration of disaster to receive assistance.[47] The Robert T. Stafford Disaster Relief and Emergency Assistance Act, PL 100-707 was signed into law November 23, 1988 and remains in effect today. This law amended the Disaster Relief Act of 1974 PL-93-288 and constitutes the statutory authority for most federal disaster response activities, especially as they pertain to the Federal Emergency Management Agency (FEMA) and FEMA programs. Although this law has been amended several times throughout the past few years, the primary purpose remains the same: to provide orderly and systematic assistance to local governments in areas of declared disaster so they can provide aid to citizens.[47]

During the Bush administration, the directives that were used to disseminate presidential decisions on national security matters were designated as National Security Presidential Directives.[48] The United States Department of Homeland Security requires states to assume an all-hazards approach to the development of competencies to prevent, prepare for, respond to, and recover from a broad array of disasters. These laws are designated as Homeland Security Presidential Directives, and stipulate continuity requirements for all executive departments and agencies. The laws provide guidance for state, local, territorial, and tribal governments, as well as private sector organizations, to ensure a comprehensive integrated national program that will enhance the credibility of the United States national security position and enable a rapid and effective response to and recovery from national emergencies.[48] Homeland Security Presidential Directive 8 establishes policies to strengthen the preparedness of the United States to prevent and respond to all disasters, and establishes mechanisms for improved delivery of preparedness assistance to federal, state, and local entities. Nurses' input into these policies is unknown.[49]

HOSPITAL EMERGENCY POLICY

Although hospitals are but one component of health care during disasters, they are critical entities during disaster response. There is a paucity of research in the literature that directly relates to nursing and hospital policy. Hospital policy is guided by standards set forth by The Joint Commission (TJC).[46] The TJC is an independent, not-for-profit organization that completes reviews, and evaluates and accredits hospitals and other health care organizations, basing its decisions on national quality and safety standards. According to TJC, hospital emergency policies should include disaster incidents both human-made and natural that are specific to the organization. Types of disasters that should be included in hospital policies are identified by probability and frequency of incidents for the area, and are based on definitions provided by the ARC and the Disaster Relief Act of 1974.

Using an exploratory, descriptive design, French and colleagues[12] investigated the needs and concerns of the nurses who responded during Hurricane Floyd. The purpose of the study was to determine whether the written plans of 4 hospitals addressed the needs and concerns of the nurses who worked during this disaster. A sample of 30 nurses who worked in the emergency department of the 4 hospitals participated in focus groups to discuss their experiences. Findings revealed that hospital policies were inadequate to deal with valid concerns of nurses. According to French and colleagues,[12] nurses' concerns included personal safety, family safety, and provision of basic needs, wages, adequate leadership, and pet care. Furthermore, the study reported that family commitment conflicted with professional obligations, resulting in nurses losing their jobs if they were unable to report to work.

Bartley and colleagues[50] completed an anonymous pre- and postinterventional study to test the hypothesis that an audiovisual presentation of hospital disaster plans would improve the knowledge, confidence, and skill of hospital employees. The sample included a convenience sample of 50 hospital employees that consisted of nurses, physicians, and administrators who would most likely be in a position of authority during a disaster. Findings showed a significant increase in the test pass-rate results from preintervention (18%) to postintervention (50%). In addition, pretest mean scores were higher for emergency room staff (12.1) versus other staff (6.2) in various areas of the hospital. The researchers also reported that there were no significant results in the general perception of preparedness. Bartley and colleagues[50] reported that the participants described the exercise as beneficial to themselves and their departments. It was acknowledged that the convenience sampling technique used to complete this study may have added to bias of the study, and that the small sample size resulted in decreased power of the study. This study suggests that simulation exercises can enhance staff knowledge levels related to disaster planning. However, it is recognized by many that more research is needed in the area of hospital disaster preparedness plans and policies.

SUMMARY

A plethora of information exists in the literature regarding emergencies and disasters. Nevertheless, significant gaps in the science related to nurses working during disasters are revealed. Few studies have addressed the perspective of nurses and their intent to respond to future disasters. Because nurses are invaluable to disaster response efforts, more research is essential to validate current findings and elucidate the needs of nurses who respond to disasters and other health emergencies.

There is a paucity of research in the literature describing nurses' lived experiences of working during hurricanes. Natural disasters inevitably inflict human suffering, and nurses are expected to respond and provide services during these catastrophic times. Lost within this expectation are the experiences and concerns of the nurses who are called upon and intend to respond to the disaster, and yet are themselves affected by the disaster. Understanding the experiences and needs of nurses who decide to respond to the call of duty and work during disasters remains unclear in the literature. Research in the area of disaster response intentions by nurses becomes the initial step in understanding the phenomenon of working during a disaster and creating innovative approaches that address working during disasters.

Disaster policies have been developed and implemented at the international, national, state, local, and hospital level. Nevertheless, disasters continue to adversely impact communities and hospitals at all levels causing injuries, death, and destruction of infrastructure. To reduce the impact of disasters, continued research is needed to inform and strengthen future disaster policies. Knowledge gained from future research has great potential to inform nursing education, research, and practice, as well as health policy related to the care of individuals and responders before, during, and after disasters.

REFERENCES

1. Agency for Healthcare Research and Quality. Surge capacity—education and training for a qualified workforce. 2004. Pub. No. 04-P028. Available at: http://archive.ahrq.gov/news/ulp/btbriefs/btbrief7.htm. Accessed January 20, 2010.
2. Agency for Healthcare Research and Quality. Bioterrorism and health system preparedness: addressing surge capacity in a mass casualty event. 2006. Pub. No. 06-0027. Available at: http://archive.ahrq.gov/news/ulp/btbriefs/btbrief9.htm. Accessed January 20, 2010.
3. Balicer R, Omer S, Barnett D, et al. Local public health perceptions toward responding to an influenza pandemic. BMC Public Health 2006;6:99.
4. Morse S, Merrill J. First steps: a pilot preparedness program for public health nurses. Mailman School of Public Health: Center for Public Health Preparedness; 2001. Available at: http://www.ncdp.mailman.columbia.edu/files/web-promo-article.pdf. Accessed September 20, 2008.
5. National Association of Public Hospitals and Health Systems. Hospital staffing and surge capacity during a disaster event. Research Brief. 2007. Available at: http://www.naph.org/naph/publications/HospitalStaffingAndSurgeCapacityDuringADisasterEvent.pdf. Accessed September 20, 2009.
6. Veenema T, editor. Disaster nursing and emergency preparedness for chemical, biological, and radiological terrorism and other hazards. 2nd edition. New York: Springer; 2007. p. 43–4, 53, 58.
7. American Red Cross. Disaster Services Connection #182. Change in the official definition of "Disaster" and the addition of a definition of "Community Emergency". 2003. Available at: http://dutchesscounty.redcross.org/Documents/182%20Community%20Emergency.pdf. Accessed January 25, 2010.
8. Giarratano G, Orlando S, Savage J. Perinatal nursing in uncertain times: the Katrina effect. MCN Am J Matern Child Nurs 2008;33(4):249–57.
9. Hughes F, Grigg M, Fritsch K, et al. Psychosocial response in emergency situations-the nurse's role. Int Nurs Rev 2007;54(1):19–27.
10. Broussard L, Myers R, Meaux J. The impact of Hurricane Katrina and Rita on Louisiana School Nurses. J Sch Nurs 2008;24(2):78–82.
11. Frank D, Sullivan L. The lived experience of nurses providing care to victims of the 2005 hurricanes. South Online J Nurs Res 2008;8(3). Available at: http://www.snrs.org/publications/SOJNR_articles2/Vol08Num03Art07.html. Accessed January 25, 2010.

12. French E, Sole M, Byers J. A comparison of nurses' needs concerns and hospital disaster plans following Florida's Hurricane Floyd. J Emerg Nurs 2002;28(2): 111–7.

13. O'Boyle C, Robertson C, Secor-Turner M. Nurses' beliefs about public health emergencies: fear of abandonment. Am J Infect Control 2006;34:351–7.

14. Brodie M, Weltzein E, Altman D, et al. Experiences of Hurricane Katrina evacuees in Houston shelters: implications for future planning. Am J Public Health 2006;96: 1402–8.

15. Slepski L. Emergency preparedness and professional competency among health care providers during hurricanes Katrina and Rita: pilot study results. Disaster Manag Response 2007;5:99–110.

16. International Nursing Coalition for Mass Casualty Education. Educational competencies for registered nurses responding to mass casualty incidents. 2003. Available at: http://www.nursing.vanderbilt.edu/incmce/competencies.html. Accessed December 15, 2009.

17. American Nurses Association. Code of ethics for nurses with interpretive statements. Washington, DC: ANA Publications; 2005. Available at: http://nursingworld. org/ethics/code/protected_nwcoe813.htm. Accessed December 15, 2009.

18. American Nurses Association. ANA comments on nursing care. 2006. Available at: http://nursingworld.org/FunctionalMenuCategories/MediaResources/PressReleases/2006/PR0927068565.aspx. Accessed January 25, 2010.

19. Nursing: scope and standards of practice. draft for public comment. 2nd edition. Silver Spring (MD): American Nurses Association; 2010. Available at. http:// nursingworld.org/DocumentVault/NursingPractice/Draft-Nursing-Scope-Standards-2nd-Ed.aspx. Accessed January 25, 2010.

20. American Association of Colleges of Nursing. The essentials of baccalaureate education. 2009. Available at: http://www.aacn.nche.edu/Education/pdf/BaccEssentials08.pdf. Accessed January 20, 2010.

21. National League for Nursing - Council of Associate Degree Nursing Competencies Task Force. Educational competencies for graduates of associate degree nursing programs. Sudbury (MA): Jones and Bartlett Publishers and National League for Nursing; 2000.

22. Gebbie K, Qureshi K. A historical challenge: nurses and emergencies. Online J Issues Nurs 2006;11(3). Manuscript 1. Available at: http://www.nursingworld. org/ojin/MainMenuCategories/ANAMarketplace/ANAPeriodicals/OJIN/TableofContents/Volume112006/Number3/NURESANDEMERGENCIES. aspx. Accessed January 20, 2010.

23. Jennings-Saunders A, Frisch N, Wing S. Nursing student's perceptions about disaster nursing. Disaster Manag Response 2005;3:80–5.

24. Weiner E, Irwin M, Trangenstein P, et al. Emergency preparedness curriculum in nursing schools in the United States. Nurs Educ Perspect 2005;26:334–9.

25. Wynd CA. Proposed model for military disaster nursing. Online J Issues Nurs 2006;11. Available at: http://www.nursingworld.org/MainMenuCategories/ANAMarketplace/ANAPeriodicals/OJIN/TableofContents/Volume112006/No3Sept06/tpc31_416085.aspx. Accessed December 15, 2009.

26. Norman E. We band of angels: the untold story of American nurses trapped on Bataan by the Japanese. New York: Pocket Books a division of Simon & Schuster, Inc; 1999.

27. Baker R, Menard S, Johns L. The military nurse experience in Vietnam: stress and impact. J Clin Psychol 1989;45:736–44.

28. Ravella P. A survey of U.S. Air Force flight nurses' adaptation to service in Vietnam. Aviat Space Environ Med 1995;66:80–3.

29. Stanton P, Dittmar S, Jezewski M, et al. Shared experiences and meaning of military nurse veterans. Image J Nurs Sch 1996;28:343–7.
30. Conner K, Foa E, Davidson J. Practical assessment and evaluation of mental health problems following mass disaster. J Clin Psychiatry 2006;67(Suppl 2): 26–33.
31. National Institute of Mental Health What is post traumatic stress disorder? 2010. Available at: http://www.nimh.nih.gov/health/topics/post-traumatic-stress-disorder-ptsd/index.shtml. Accessed July 15, 2010.
32. United States Department of Veterans Affairs. National center for PTSD: advancing science and promoting understanding of traumatic stress. 2010. Available at: http://www.ptsd.va.gov/. Accessed July 15, 2010.
33. Lerner M, Shelton R. Acute traumatic stress management: addressing emergent psychological needs during traumatic events. New York: The American Academy of Experts in Traumatic Stress; 2001.
34. Cardeña E, Speigel D. Dissociative reactions to the San Francisco Bay Area earthquake of 1989. Am J Psychiatry 1993;150:474–8.
35. Koopman C, Classen C, Spiegel D. Predictors of posttraumatic stress symptoms among survivors of the Oakland/Berkeley, California firestorm. Am J Psychiatry 1994;151:888–94.
36. Breslau N, Davis GC, Andreski P, et al. Sex differences in posttraumatic stress disorder. Arch Gen Psychiatry 1997;54:1044–8.
37. Laposa JM, Alden LE, Fullerton L. Work stress and post-traumatic stress disorder in the emergency department. J Emerg Nurs 2003;29:23–9.
38. Brewin C, Rose S, Andrews B, et al. Brief screening instrument for post-traumatic stress disorder. Br J Psychiatry 2002;181:158–62.
39. Qureshi K, Gershon R, Sherman M, et al. Health care workers' ability and willingness to report to duty during catastrophic disasters. J Urban Health 2005;82(3): 378–88.
40. Ruderman C, Tracy C, Bensimon C, et al. On pandemic and the duty to care: whose duty? Who cares? BMC Med Ethics 2006;7:E5.
41. Ehrenstein B, Hanses F, Salzberger B. Influenza pandemic and professional duty: family or patients first? A survey of hospital employees. BMC Public Health 2006; 6:311.
42. Grimes D, Mendias E. Nurses' intentions to respond to bioterrorism and other infectious disease emergencies. Nurs Outlook 2010;58:10–6.
43. James N, Miller C, Nugent K, et al. The impact of Hurricane Katrina on older adult nurses: an assessment of quality of life and psychological distress in the aftermath. J Miss State Med Assoc 2007;48:299–307.
44. Polit D, Beck S. Nursing research: principles and methods. 8th edition. Philadelphia: Lippincott; 2008.
45. Sullivent E III, West C, Noe S, et al. Nonfatal injuries following hurricane Katrina—New Orleans Louisiana 2005. J Safety Res 2006;37:213–7.
46. The Joint Commission Emergency management. 2010. Available at: http://www.jointcommission.org/AccreditationPrograms/Hospitals/Standards/09_FAQs/EM/Emergency_Management.htm. Accessed July 20, 2010.
47. Federal Emergency Management Agency. Robert T. Stafford Disaster Relief and Emergency Assistance Act, as amended and Related 2007.
48. United States Department of Homeland Security. Homeland Security Presidential Directive 5: management of domestic incidents. 2003. Available at: http://www.dhs.gov/xabout/laws/gc_1214592333605.shtm. Accessed December 15, 2009.

49. Federal Emergency Management Agency Declared disasters by year and state. 2008. Available at: http://www.fema.gov/news/disaster_totals_annual.fema. Accessed December 15, 2009.

50. Bartley B, Stella J, Walsh L. What a disaster? Assessing utility of simulated disaster exercise and associated educational process. Prehospital Disaster Med 2006;21:249–55.

Financial and Economic Considerations for Emergency Response Providers

Anne S. Liong, PhD, MBA, RN[a],*, Samuel U. Liong, MS, MBA, RN, PMP[b]

KEYWORDS

- Financial • Economic • Emergency response providers
- First responders

Traditionally, the term first responders referred to local police, firefighters, and emergency medical personnel who provided an immediate response to crises on site. In light of concerns about bioterrorism and other potential terrorist attacks, the Homeland Security Act of 2002 broadened the scope of first responders to include "federal, state, and local emergency, public safety, law enforcement, emergency response, emergency medical (including hospital emergency facilities), and related personnel, agencies, and authorities."[1] Now referred to as emergency response providers, these groups are responsible for the protection and preservation of life, property, evidence, as well as the environment in the early stages of an incident.[2]

First responders put their lives at risk everyday to serve communities. Therefore, financial support to fund planning, exercises, and interoperable communication systems; facilitating the establishment of standards and guidelines; and integrating best practices to prepare for disasters are imperative. Emergency response providers need to be afforded with commensurate compensation, benefits, and protection to safeguard their welfare as well as assure support to their dependents and survivors if an injury, a permanent disability, or even death occurs. In addition, incentives and recognition encourage emergency response provider participation and promotion of recruitment efforts that help to build and sustain more resilient emergency response provider communities throughout the country.

The authors have nothing to disclose.
[a] Nursing Standards and Policies, Nursing Practice and Professional Advancement, Harris County Hospital District, 5656 Kelley, Houston, TX 77026, USA
[b] School of Biomedical Informatics, University of Texas Health Science Center at Houston, 7000 Fannin, Houston, TX 77030, USA
* Corresponding author. Harris County Hospital District, 1504 Taub Loop, Houston, TX 77030.
E-mail address: anne_liong@hchd.tmc.edu

CHANNELING THE DOLLARS

To safeguard the welfare of these special groups of people who assume key roles at critical times, financial and economic factors need to be considered. In the United States, the federal government has been charged with awarding grants; providing planning, training, and exercises; establishing standards and guidelines; and providing compensation and benefits to first responders and their families.

The critical nature of the need for high-tech communication was one of the vulnerabilities identified during the terrorist attacks on the World Trade Center (WTC) on September 11, 2001. The inability to communicate across providers and jurisdictions was evident in a court-ordered release of the New York City Fire Department radio communications that revealed 15 hours of panic, confusion, and frustration. According to Congressman Bart Stupak (D-MI), "With more than 80 percent of America's local first responders not able to interoperate or communicate with their counterparts, the inability of first responders to communicate with each other is more than a major concern; it's a threat to our national security."[3]

Streamlining grant assistance process through the enactment of laws is important to first responders. It gives them access to funds through less cumbersome and circuitous methods. In addition, it also helps allocate the grants to places where the need and risks are high. The Faster and Smarter Funding for First Responders Acts (H.R. 3266 in 2003 and H.R. 1544 in 2005) were proposed to increase the efficiency in providing grant assistance to first responders. H.R. 3266 specified the need for an expert task force that would advise the Secretary of Homeland Security on the capabilities that different communities should prepare for potential terrorist attacks to fund actual needs.[4]

In addition, the bill proposed that regions with shared needs apply for homeland security grants as well as the preservation of all pre-9/11 federal grants available to support first responders. H.R. 1544 had similar purposes. The administration supported it but several concerns were raised regarding the specific allocation of funds, the Department of Homeland Security (DHS) grant review process, and the new oversight requirements.[5] Unfortunately, these bills never came to fruition.

Although it is important to address current issues, it is equally vital to drive an efficient funding process for a unique group of individuals providing critical services during catastrophic events. The Government Accountability Office reviewed the states that received grants between 2003 and 2005, and the report showed that strategic plans to allocate funds were not generally used to guide investments on appropriate tools.[6] One such tool is a disaster communication system. This is a system that is composed of communication devices, processes, protocols, and a universal language, in which feedback loops are easily understood by first responders coming from disparate sectors, professions, or locations.

In 2010, the Federal Emergency Management Agency (FEMA) was awarded with more than $1.8 billion for preparedness grants for the fiscal year 2010.[7] The grants provide the first responder community with funds to conduct planning, exercises, and training. The funding also helps to pay for the purchase of equipment necessary for the first responders' role. This equipment includes communication devices enhanced with interoperable features to improve coordination efforts during disasters.

PLANNING AND EXERCISES

Preparing for a disaster involves creating a project management plan that has an undefined execution date. Mock disasters are created, and the plan goes through trial runs to evaluate it. Federal government programs set the stage for successful preparation of the first responder group. The Homeland Security Exercise and Evaluation Program (HSEEP) provided a national standard for the methodology and terminology of exercise design, development, conduct, evaluation, and improvement planning.[8] Through exercises, the National Exercise Program supports organizations to perform an objective assessment of their capabilities so that the strengths and areas for improvement are identified, corrected, and shared as appropriate, before a real incident.

Lessons learned in actual and imminent disasters should be considered and appropriately integrated during the planning stages. At the local level, a successful rapid response operation was demonstrated by Harris County in Houston, Texas, after a landfall on the Gulf Coast on August 29, 2005, caused by the Hurricane Katrina. The hurricane, which killed 1836 people, was one of the costliest and deadliest natural disasters in US history. The breach of the levee system in New Orleans and other hurricane-related damage resulted in the evacuation of as many as 373,000 Gulf Coast residents.[9] A large number of sick and injured evacuees were transported to Houston's Astrodome/Reliant Center Complex. The Regional Hospital Preparedness Council's Catastrophic Medical Operations Center was activated, and a triage plan was developed for arriving evacuees. A 2009 report documented the challenges of the response efforts and offered 5 recommendations: (1) implementation of an evacuee tracking system, (2) use of integrated patient medical record systems, (3) use of waste management/hygiene facilities, (4) availability of transportation within the shelter facilities for evacuees, and (5) use of communication networks during disasters.[10]

Several strategies that were used ensured the successful evacuation of the University of Texas Medical Branch at Galveston in September 2005, during the threat of Hurricane Rita, a category 5 storm, which initially aimed for the Houston-Galveston area.[11] Factors that were considered crucial for success, such as leadership, communication, transportation, partnership, and prioritizing patient safety, were identified. Recommendations were also made to help develop more efficient systems and processes and improve patient outcomes for future disaster response.

STANDARDS, GUIDELINES, AND BEST PRACTICES

The FEMA "supports our citizens and first responders to ensure that as a nation we work together to build, sustain, and improve our capability to prepare for, protect against, respond to, recover from, and mitigate all hazards."[12] Several entities under FEMA work closely to provide standards and guidelines for disaster management. The National Response Framework provides the structure and mechanisms for the national-level policy for incident management. The National Incident Management System (NIMS) establishes the framework and processes to guide departments at all levels of government, nongovernmental organizations, and the private sector to coordinate response and recovery efforts. The National Integration Center publishes the standards, guidelines, and compliance protocols for determining whether a federal, state, tribal, or local government has implemented NIMS. The standards, policies, and guidelines offer first responders a certain level of assurance that disaster management activities are organized and standardized. However, questions prevail regarding adherence to such standards and guidelines and compliance to policies by all groups involved in actual disaster responses.

Emergency response providers based in hospitals (also called first receivers) risk their health as well as their lives while performing their jobs. The Occupational Safety and Health Administration developed and published a best practices document for facilities that receive mass casualty incidents involving the release of hazardous substances. The document contains useful information including victim decontamination, personal protective equipment, and employee training to prevent or mitigate the effects of hazardous material exposure.[13]

COMPENSATION, BENEFITS, AND PROTECTIONS

Volunteer medical groups, such as the Disaster Medical Assistance Teams (DMATs), are paid while serving as part-time federal employees.[14] Activated DMAT personnel are appointed to an appropriate federal status and a corresponding pay rate. Team members with specific expertise and experience within a wide range of professions are recruited through the National Disaster Medical System (NDMS). The NDMS/DMAT personnel are required to maintain appropriate certifications and licensure within their discipline. When personnel are activated as federal employees, all states recognize their licensure and certification. The Federal Tort Claims Act protects the DMAT personnel in the event of malpractice claims.

DMATs deploy to disaster sites with sufficient supplies and equipment to sustain themselves for a period of 72 hours, while providing medical care at a fixed or temporary medical care site until other federal or contract resources are mobilized or the situation is resolved. Personnel are activated for a period of 2 weeks. In mass casualty incidents, their responsibilities may include triaging patients, providing high-quality medical care despite the adverse environment that is often typical of a disaster site, patient reception at staging facilities, and preparing patients for evacuation. The responder's primary (full-time, non-NDMS) employment is protected for approved training and deployment under the Uniformed Services Employment and Reemployment Rights Act as long as the volunteer meets the eligibility requirements. The Public Health System (PHS) provides transportation, food supplies, shelter, and logistic support to the DMAT. The PHS is responsible for compensating DMAT members for expenses incurred during the performance of their assigned tasks and transporting them back after the completion of the emergency incident. Members who are injured anytime during the deployment phase are entitled to federal employee benefits such as medical insurance and workman's compensation.

OTHER COMPENSATIONS FOR INJURED WORKERS AND SURVIVORS

During the immediate and recovery periods of the WTC attacks in 2001, a large number of people, including first responders, were exposed to harmful particulate matter. The area was enveloped in a thick plume of smoke that contained cement dust, glass fibers, asbestos, lead, hydrochloric acid, polychlorinated biphenyls, and organochlorine pesticides.[15–18] The federal September 11th Victim Compensation Fund previously paid more than $7 billion in public compensation to the families of those who died in the WTC attacks and to the injured survivors.[19] A portion of the amount ($500 million) went to more than 1300 recovery workers and others suffering from respiratory injuries. More first responders and other workers reported new and worsening respiratory symptoms and illnesses. However, many workers had not visited health care providers regularly before 9/11, and there was no reliable method to determine when their respiratory symptoms and illnesses began.[20] Controversy stemming from the 9/11 research and reports resulted in lawsuits filed by 10,000 plaintiffs who suffered respiratory and other illnesses. A recent report indicated that a new settlement was reached, adding $55.5 million to the original amount ($657 million).[21] The payout is likely to increase by as much as $125 million to those injured by the harmful dust.

BENEFITS AND SCHOLARSHIPS

Other benefits and scholarships are available to first responders and their families. The federal Public Safety Officers Benefits program was recently extended to first responders who work or volunteer for nonprofit organizations.[22,23] This extension of the program removes the delineation between federal government, state government, local government, or nonprofit agency affiliations. If first responders are permanently disabled or killed, benefits are paid to eligible survivors. This benefit is adjusted each federal fiscal year to reflect the percentage of change in the consumer price index. For each death and disability claim, the award amount is determined by the actual date of the person's death or disability. As of October 1, 2008, the benefit is $315,764.

Scholarship funds (Families of Freedom Scholarship Fund) provide need-based postsecondary scholarships to qualified members of the 9/11 community. The community includes the financially eligible dependents of those people killed or permanently disabled in the WTC terrorist attacks as well as during the rescue activities related to the incidents. Since 2002, when the scholarships were first distributed, more than $49 million was awarded to approximately 1452 students.[24] The fund will continue to provide educational assistance till 2030, and will provide $10.5 million to affected family members and relief workers in school year 2010-2011, including 173 first-time recipients.

At present, personal income tax credits are being offered by several states to first responders. For example, Pennsylvania provides up to $100 and New York State offers $200 for eligible first responders.[25] Some states have pending proposals to increase the credit up to $1000 per year. Other states provide alternative real personal property tax exemption through local municipalities.

INCENTIVES

Private employers provide bonuses to staff who work during disasters. In 2001, Tropical Storm Allison resulted in about 3 ft of rain over several days in Houston, Texas. It produced massive flooding and caused power outage in the Texas Medical Center area. Among the institutions that were severely affected were The Methodist Hospital and Memorial Hermann Hospital. Despite the financial losses, both the hospitals gave the "flood heroes" bonuses and recognition. In 2005, The Methodist Hospital also gave gift cards and extra hours in paid-time-off bank to the employees who helped prepare for Hurricane Rita.[26] Fortunately, the hurricane veered away from Houston at the last minute and spared the city. According to the hospital system's employee relations director, "It's a small gesture to let employees know they're valued and appreciated." Home builders and lenders have also strongly expressed their readiness to helping first responders by offering incentives such as discounts and special concessions toward the purchase of a home.

IMPLICATIONS TO NURSES AND NURSE LEADERS

During disasters, nurses often participate as volunteered first responders (ie, DMAT) or as first receivers in emergency hospitals. In both cases, nurses need to maintain licensure and certification, participate in necessary training and exercises, stay cognizant of best practices, and comply with applicable laws, policies, and standards. Nurses should be aware of financial and other support resources that are available through the government and the private sector. Nurses who want to help during disasters can volunteer through NDMS or other private organizations such as the Red Cross.

Nurse leaders in hospitals manage the largest staff group, with nursing care often the costliest item in the budget. Because the preparation for disaster management requires expenditures, nurse leaders must scan the environment for grant opportunities at all levels as well as develop creative ways to complete staff training and education. Moreover, it is important that nurse leaders are able to determine costs, direct allocation, and advocate expenses to effectively manage scarce resources. Nurse executives must work to integrate disaster planning into all areas of clinical decision making. Nurse leaders need to be aware of information regarding staff needs during disasters, such as financial compensation, policies addressing work assignments, flexibility for extenuating circumstances, pet care, family sheltering, and provision of basic needs.[27]

Nurse leaders with experience in managing disasters should share their information so that other leaders may learn and develop improved disaster response processes applicable to their organizations. In addition, proactive efforts should increase the sharing of information in order to reach legislators, so that the outcomes of disaster response decisions can guide policy makers.

SUMMARY

Catastrophic events often threaten or cause depletion of resources. It is generally accepted that changes inherent to disasters are stressful. The Conservation of Resources Theory predicts that positive and negative changes in resources will have markedly different effects.[28] This theory proposes that resource losses are psychologically stressful, whereas resource gains buffer against the effects of resource loss.

For first responders, the level of preparedness is crucial. Investments in planning, training, and logistics are necessary to mitigate the stress associated with a crisis. Stress is also related to not knowing the future of their loved ones if death or permanent incapacity occurs, hence specific laws and financial resources provide a safety net to dependents of first responders and survivors. This kind of safety gives the first responders peace of mind and assurance that the future of their dependents will not be jeopardized. Incentives that are offered let the first responders know that they are valued and appreciated.

Indeed, financial support considerably helps first responders before, during, and after catastrophic events. It assists them to cope with stress at the individual level and allows them to become more resilient; this resonates to the community and country in which they serve and enhances their potential to save lives and prevent disabilities.

REFERENCES

1. Department of Homeland Security. Homeland Security Act of 2002. Available at: http://www.dhs.gov/xabout/laws/law_regulation_rule_0011.shtm. Accessed June 1, 2010.
2. Homeland Security Presidential Directive 8. National preparedness. Available at: http://www.fas.org/irp/offdocs/nspd/hspd-8.html. Accessed June 1, 2010.
3. Michigan's 1st District: News from Congressman Bart Stupak. 9–11 tapes reveal communication chaos, stupak stresses need for first responder interoperability, August 15, 2005. 2005. Available at: http://www.house.gov/list/press/mi01_stupak/081505interop.html. Accessed June 10, 2010.
4. Homeland Security. Chairman Christopher Cox: HR 3266 faster and smarter funding for first responders commonly asked questions. 2003. Available at: http://

www.iwar.org.uk/homesec/resources/hsas-hearing/10-15-03-1ST-Rspdr-QA11.pdf. Accessed June 13, 2010.

5. The White House. Statement of administration policy: HR 1544 faster and smarter funding for first responders of 2005. 2002. Available at: http://www.whitehouse. gov/sites/default/files/omb/assets/omb/legislative/sap/109-1/hr1544sap-h.pdf. Accessed June 7, 2010.

6. Government Accountability Office. Report to congressional requesters: first responders much work remains to improve communications interoperability (April 2007). Available at: http://www.gao.gov/new.items/d07301.pdf. Accessed June 7, 2010.

7. Department of Homeland Security. Secretary Napolitano announces more than $1.8 billion in fiscal year 2010 preparedness grants. July 15, 2010. Available at: http://www.dhs.gov/ynews/releases/pr_1279205905487.shtm. Accessed June 3, 2010.

8. Homeland Security Exercise and Evaluation Program. HSEEP mission. 2010. Available at: https://hseep.dhs.gov/pages/1001_HSEEP7.aspx. Accessed May 16, 2010.

9. United States Senate. Statement of Robert A. Eckels, County Judge, Harris County, Texas before the Senate Homeland Security and Governmental Affairs Committee hearing on recovering from Hurricane Katrina: responding to the needs of the displaced, today and tomorrow. Available at: http://www.harriscountycitizencorps. com/newsletters/raetestimony.pdf. Accessed May 27, 2010.

10. Hamilton DR, Gavagan TF, Smart KT, et al. Houston's medical disaster response to Hurricane Katrina: part 1: the initial medical response from Trauma Service Area Q. Ann Emerg Med 2009;53(4):505–14.

11. Sexton KH, Alperin LM, Stobo JD. Lessons learned from Hurricane Rita University of Texas medical branch hospital's evacuation. Acad Med 2007;82(8):792–6.

12. Federal Emergency Management Agency. FEMA mission. 2010. Available at: http://www2.fema.gov/about/index.shtm. Accessed May 3, 2010.

13. Occupational Safety and Health Administration. Best practices for hospital-based first receivers of victims from mass casualty incidents involving the release of hazardous substances. 2005. Available at: http://osha.gov/dts/osta/bestpractices/html/hospital_firstreceivers.html. Accessed June 13, 2010.

14. National Disaster Medical System. Disaster medical assistance team. 2010. Available at: http://www.phe.gov/Preparedness/responders/ndms/teams/Pages/dmat.aspx. Accessed May 25, 2010.

15. Clark RN, Green RO, Sayze GA, et al. Environmental studies of the world trade center area after the September 11, 2001 attacks. 2003. Available at: http://pubs.usgs.gov/of/2001/ofr-01-0429. Accessed June 30, 2010.

16. Landrigan PJ, Lioy PJ, Thurston G, et al. Health and environmental consequences of the world trade center disaster. Environ Health Perspect 2004;112(6):731–9.

17. Lioy PJ, Weisel CP, Milette JR, et al. Characterization of dust/smoke aerosol that settled east of the World Trade Center (WTC) in lower Manhattan after the collapse of the WTC 11 September 2001. Environ Health Perspect 2002;110(7):703–14.

18. McGee JK, Chen LC, Cohen MD, et al. Chemical analysis of world trade center fine particulate matter for use in toxicologic assessment. Environ Health Perspect 2003;11(7):972–80.

19. Pak VM, O'Hara ME, McCauley LA. Health effects following 9/11. AAOHN J 2008; 56(4):159–65.

20. DePalma A, Kovaleski SF. Accuracy of 9/11 health reports is questioned. Available at: http://www.nytimes.com/2007/09/07/nyregion/07sinai.html?_r=1. Accessed June 5, 2010.
21. Hamblett M. New settlement reached in 9/11 injury cases. 2010. Available at: http://www.law.com/jsp/article.jsp?id=1202462596084. Accessed July 3, 2010.
22. Federal Benefits for Public Safety Officers. Available at: http://www.statetroopers.org/PDFs/FedBens.pdf. Accessed June 1, 2010.
23. Fireburg H. Federal death benefits extended to emsEMS personnel. 2009. Available at: http://www.usfra.org/emsforum/topics/federal-death-benefits#axzz0x ENGFiaa. Accessed May 18, 2010.
24. Families of Freedom Scholarship Fund. Families of freedom will provide $10.5 million to 9/11 family members & relief workers in 2010-2011. 2010. Available at: http://www.familiesoffreedom.org/. Accessed June 15, 2010.
25. VanDeCarr J. Volunteer firefighter personal income tax credit law. 2008. Available at: http://www.fasny.com/pdfs/VolFireIncomeTax.pdf. Accessed May 27, 2010.
26. Ladika S. HR magazine. 2006. Available at: http://findarticles.com/p/articles/mi_m3495/is_9_51/ai_n26993585/. Accessed June 30, 2010.
27. French ED, Sole ML, Byers JF. A comparison of nurses' needs/concerns and hospital disaster plans following Florida's hurricane Floyd. J Emerg Nurs 2002; 28(2):111–7.
28. Hobfall SE, Schumm JA. Conservation of Resources Theory. In: Diclemente RJ, Crosby RA, Kegler MC, editors. Emerging theories in health promotion practice and research. San Francisco (CA): Jossey-Bass; 2002. p. 287–8.

Physical and Environmental Considerations for First Responders

Karen S. Migl, PhD, RNC, WHNP-BC[a],*, Rose M. Powell, PhD, RN[b]

KEYWORDS

• Disaster • Physical • Environmental • First responders

Disasters are by their very nature problematic in that they arrive unexpectedly and in most cases, without warning. Postdisaster intervention requires coordinating complex recovery efforts because of the massive extent of disruption of services, displacement of people, and interrupted or disabled communication. Health care professionals find themselves in unique situations, making decisions regarding administering care or providing services, given the unusual circumstances or events. The decisions that responders make are affected by the resources that are available, the unusual practice settings, and the lack of familiarity with precise patient care needs.

The American Nurses Association (ANA) has attempted to respond to the questions that nurses have raised regarding the standards of care under extreme conditions such as disasters, pandemics, earthquakes, and other extreme emergencies. While the ANA has suggested guidelines for health care professionals during disasters, pandemics, and other extreme emergencies, the 2 most important recommendations are to maintain a state of professional readiness for emergency response and to plan for and practice emergency response.[1]

There are many physical and environmental issues that health care providers (HCP) as first responders must consider when dealing with disasters. Human response to a disaster is different for each individual. For first responders, possessing a foundation of factual information depending on the type of disaster is of critical importance for HCPs to aid in the healing process in ways they think are effective.

This work was not supported by any funding.
The authors have nothing to disclose.
[a] RN-BSN Online Track, Richard and Lucille DeWitt School of Nursing, Stephen F. Austin State University, PO Box 6156, Stephen F. Austin Station, Nacogdoches, TX 75962, USA
[b] Leadership in Nursing Systems, Richard and Lucille DeWitt School of Nursing, Stephen F. Austin State University, PO Box 6156, Stephen F. Austin Station, Nacogdoches, TX 75962, USA
* Corresponding author.
E-mail address: kmigl@sfasu.edu

This article examines the physical and environmental issues that health care professionals in the role of first responders may encounter during disasters or extreme emergencies. It is hoped that discussing this issue will help health care professionals to gain an understanding of the physical and environmental considerations during disasters and therefore to provide the care needed for healing and recovery for both their patients and themselves.

HUMAN RESPONSE

It is important to understand that the history of worldwide disasters, both natural and human-made, have given global, national, state, regional, and local communities an improved insight into the need for disaster mitigation. This process is ongoing, and after a disaster response, there is a continued imperative to learn and make improvements from the lessons learned from each event, analyzing the effectiveness of the response to better prepare for the next event.[2]

Whereas first responders may well understand the process of triage during disasters, they may not be familiar with dealing with mass casualties. HCPs may feel overwhelmed at the sight of dead bodies in disaster situations. It is important for them to know that there is little evidence to suggest that cadavers pose a risk for disease in areas where the disease is not endemic. One of the deadliest earthquakes in Turkey's history occurred in August 1999, causing 16,000 deaths and 44,000 injuries. A study conducted after the earthquake revealed that emergency teams that came to the earthquake site first dealt with the emergency and then the treatment process. The emergency teams treated immediate injuries, illnesses, and traumas resulting from the earthquake. Most of the treatment consisted of surgery, childbirth, trauma, and neonatal and postneonatal care. The emergency teams saw little infectious disease and prioritized their efforts on searching for survivors, treatment and care of the injured, and management of the displaced survivors. The disposal of the dead was not a priority during this time because the concern was to save and treat the injured.[3]

In contrast, Haiti's earthquake on January 12, 2010 struck near the country's capital Port-au-Prince and was the strongest earthquake in country in more than 200 years. Haiti already had a high poverty population of 67%. About 1.5 million people were directly affected by the earthquake, and it is estimated that approximately 220,000 people died and more than 300,000 were injured. Haiti had a difficult time providing public health services before the earthquake, and the devastation resulting from the earthquake presented new challenges to an already desperate situation. However, the massive number of dead bodies did not add to outbreaks of disease or epidemics. It was almost 6 months before the Centers for Disease Control and Prevention (CDC) received reports of dengue fever among the relief workers returning from Haiti and issued a health advisory. Dengue fever is endemic in Haiti, and the lack of shelter and utilities such as electricity and water pose an even greater risk of the disease, becoming more widespread as the population and health care workers are exposed to the elements and opportunities for mosquito breeding grounds grow.[4,5]

In 1998, Hurricane Mitch devastated Central America and proved to be one of the most devastating and deadly hurricanes in history. There were an estimated 10000 deaths because of flooding and landslides. The flooding of roads and destruction of health centers hindered emergency relief efforts and was the immediate cause of morbidity and mortality. Initially, the emergency response teams treated a great number of the injured; however, their focus shifted as evidenced by a study of infectious diseases before and after Hurricane Mitch in the Nicaraguan community of Villanueva. Results showed that there was a significant increase in the incidence of acute diarrhea and acute respiratory tract infection.[6] The evidence suggested that the increased incidence of these illnesses was attributable to flooding, poor sanitation conditions, overcrowding, and damage to the basic infrastructure. This study was unique in that it was performed at the same time as relief operations and served to assist the relief teams in prioritization of services. There was no evidence to link the presence of dead bodies to increased rates of infection. However, lack of drinking water, poor hygiene, and overcrowding were indicated as the primary factors in the increase in the incidences of these illnesses. Findings from a study published after the hurricane stated that the devastation in Central America resulted more from economic and political policies than from natural disaster.[7] The study revealed that during the years, poorer populations had been forced from their stable farming land to degraded hillsides and into floodplains, which made these people particularly vulnerable to the effects of the hurricane. Nicaragua had an inappropriate emergency planning, which greatly exacerbated the death toll from Hurricane Mitch. The population settlements in degraded areas coupled with the failure to anticipate the disaster through massive evacuations or to respond effectively to the damages caused the loss of thousands of lives. The rescue and care of survivors in any disaster is undoubtedly of a higher priority than attending to the disposal of dead bodies.

The aforementioned examples as well as many health institutions have provided evidence that dead bodies do not present a public health hazard. The World Health Organization (WHO) has repeatedly pointed out that there is a minimal risk for infection from dead bodies. In a document published in 2002, WHO established that "[d]ead or decayed human bodies do not generally create a serious health hazard, unless they are polluting sources of drinking water with fecal matter, or are infected with plague or typhus, in which case they may be infested with the fleas or lice that spread these diseases."[8]

According to scientists from the Water, Engineering and Development Centre (WEDC), United Kingdom, the relationship between corpses and epidemics has never been scientifically demonstrated or reported. Contrary to popular belief, corpses rarely contaminate water sources and are not associated with the transmission of malaria or dengue. Most potential agents do not survive long after death, and the dead body remains only pose a public health risk in cases of death from cholera or hemorrhagic fevers. The hurried disposal of dead bodies may constitute more of a hazard for public health than the corpses themselves. For example, mass cremations produce high quantities of smoke with airborne dioxin, resulting in significant respiratory problems.[9] The experiences of the WHO and the WEDC in managing disasters in which there are large numbers of dead bodies and subsequent health-related problems supports the evidence that the presence of corpses plays a negligible role in the spread of infectious diseases. Although decaying bodies create very little risk of major disease outbreaks, risks are associated with those who handle the bodies or prepare them for burial. This evidence should be provided to HCPs, emergency workers, and the general public so that the disposal and handling of dead bodies may be appropriate. Importantly, this information and communication would help meet the grieving families' needs for social and cultural customs for end-of-life rituals and funerals as well as demonstrating respect for the survivors.[10–13]

HEALTH PROMOTION

HCPs need have knowledge of and follow recommended protocols. Primary priorities for first responders are to ensure that they are up-to-date on personal immunizations, anticipate safety issues, and are as prepared as possible. For example, the CDC recommends that when traveling to disaster areas, it is a personal responsibility to be aware of the risks and take all possible measures to minimize those risks. In traveling to assist in any disaster, there are many things that HCPs should be aware of and teach others traveling into the affected regions.[14]

Recommended Immunizations

It is the responsibility of all persons traveling into a disaster-struck area to ensure that they have received all their routine immunizations such as those for tetanus/diphtheria, polio, and measles. Some vaccines such as polio, influenza, typhoid, and measles vaccines only need to be administered in a single dose and may be given all at the same time. However, some vaccine schedules can be accelerated to help accommodate individuals trying to reach disaster areas as quickly and safely as possible. Because the possibility of infections and disease outbreaks is increased after disasters, the following vaccines are recommended by the CDC:

- Tetanus/diphtheria vaccine or booster, if the vaccine or booster was given 5 years ago or earlier
- Hepatitis A
- Hepatitis B
- Influenza
- Typhoid (oral or injectable)
- Polio, if no booster has been given since childhood
- Measles
- Rabies
- Japanese encephalitis.

Cholera
In the event of outbreaks of cholera reported in the region, cholera vaccine is recommended. However, cholera vaccine is not available in the United States, therefore first responders need to know where to obtain the vaccine and be aware that it requires time for the antibody to develop and offer protection.[15]

Yellow fever
Yellow fever vaccine is recommended for a person traveling to affected areas in East Africa. This vaccine is also mandatory for entry into certain countries in Central Africa and South America. Although there is no yellow fever risk in Asia, some countries may require documentation of yellow fever vaccination for people traveling from yellow fever endemic areas. Other countries may require proof of immunization if the travel includes a stopover in a country where yellow fever is known to exist.[16]

Malaria prophylaxis
There is no immunization against malaria, and although no antimalarial drug is 100% protective, taking antimalarial drugs correctly and consistently is the most important factor in preventing this debilitating and potentially fatal condition. Administration of antimalarial drugs should be started 1 week before departure, taken during the stay, and continued for 4 weeks after leaving the region where malaria is prevalent.

An added prophylactic measure against malaria is the use of an insecticide-treated bed net. Bed nets offer a protective barrier against the female malaria-carrying mosquitoes that are nocturnal and bite at night. Mosquito nets with an insecticide woven into the net kills and repels mosquitoes, adding protection for others who may not have a net, thus benefiting the entire community.[17]

Personal immunization considerations

- Always ensure that your immunizations are up-to-date. Keep an immunization record, with the important records in a designated safe file so that it is easily accessible. As an HCP or a first responder, it is important to ensure your own health as well as that of those with whom you are aiding in times of disaster.
- If you are traveling to an area where the sanitary conditions are poor and the drinking water is unsafe, you should receive immunizations against typhoid and hepatitis A.
- Make sure you are both properly informed and aware of the risks involved when travel involves remote areas that require meningitis, Japanese encephalitis, European tick-borne encephalitis, hepatitis B, or rabies immunizations.
- Before you travel, have your own immunizations evaluated by an expert in international travel requirements. It is also prudent to know your own physical health and any limitations, exactly where you are traveling, and the countries you must travel through to get to your destination. (This knowledge may determine some immunizations that you may need to take.)
- Although most vaccines can be administered on short notice, 4 to 6 weeks before departure is the recommended time for immunization to maximize your protection because it takes time for your body to acquire immunity.
- Immunizations offer protection against disease, but proper hand washing, personal hygiene, safe food and water sources, and precautions to prevent mosquito bites ensure personal health.[14–16]

INJURY RISKS

After a natural disaster, the risk for injury is increased. Providers anticipating traveling into a disaster area needs to make sure that they dress appropriately and wear sturdy footwear that offers protection from the widespread debris. While tetanus is a potential health threat for persons who sustain wound injuries, HCPs need to assess any wound or rash that has the potential for becoming infected. Any wound, cut, or animal bite should be immediately cleansed with soap and clean water. Evidence shows that most injuries in floods and hurricanes are caused by soft tissue injuries and cuts. Because of the circumstances, the wounds are usually heavily contaminated and require immediate attention, with prophylactic antibiotic therapy and tetanus if indicated.

Motor vehicle crashes are a leading cause of serious injury among travelers going into a disaster area. These crashes may be due in part to being unfamiliar with the local vehicle speed limits and laws. However, use of common sense can protect from motor vehicle crashes, such as avoiding drinking and driving and always wearing a safety belt. Being aware of and following the local customs and laws regarding pedestrian safety and vehicle speed are critical. In all aspects of transportation, safety should be first and foremost. The use of helmets on bicycles, motorcycles, and motor-bikes is instrumental in the prevention of injury. Although tempting during times of disaster, HCPs should refrain from boarding an overloaded bus or minibus, and whenever possible a local driver familiar with the area should be hired.[18,19]

Electrocution Prevention

During disaster there are many power outages. HCPs need to be aware of their environment and take steps to keep everyone safe. Sometimes there may be downed power lines, so it is important to treat all power lines as hot to avoid possible electrocution. Many individuals have portable generators and are competent in their proper use. However, a problem arises if the portable generator is improperly installed and operated. This improper installation and operation could cause a problem called back-feed or feedback in the power lines and could seriously injure or kill repair workers. HCPs should not attempt to operate or repair power lines or equipment with which they are unfamiliar. It may be in the best safety interest of all concerned to use battery-operated flashlight and lanterns, avoiding the use of candles or any other flame devices that could cause injury.[16,19]

Water- and Food-Borne Risks

Natural disasters contribute to the spread of many serious food and water-borne diseases, especially because water supplies and sewage systems have been disrupted. Diarrheal diseases such as typhoid, hepatitis A, and *Escherichia coli* infection can possibly be caused by contaminated water sources. Bottled water may be a convenient solution for travelers visiting countries where a disaster has occurred and there is known poor hygiene and inadequate sanitation. According to the CDC and the Environmental Protection Agency, if bottled water is not available, boiling water for 1 minute causes common intestinal pathogens to be inactivated. For disasters in the United States, boiling water is usually recommended. The most common chemical water disinfectants that are promoted by the WHO Safe Water System for individual households in developing countries are chlorine and iodine. As with other infectious illnesses, one of the most important preventive practices is careful and frequent hand washing. Cleaning hands often using either soap and water or waterless, alcohol-based hand wash removes potentially infectious materials from the skin and helps prevent disease transmission.[20,21]

Food is important during times of disaster but not as important or as critical as water. The food of choice should be easily prepared or require no preparation at all. Foods such as dry pasta, rice, vegetable oil, soybeans, and bouillon may be stored indefinitely and canned meat, vegetables, and fruits up to 1 year or according to the label expiration date. Meals ready to eat are complete meals with heaters that only require a small amount of water to activate.[19,22]

Risks from Insect Bites

During disaster, standing water may become mosquito breeding grounds, causing potential outbreaks of malaria, Japanese encephalitis, and dengue. In addition to malaria prophylaxis and Japanese encephalitis vaccine, other measures should be used for protection from mosquito and other insect bites. Using insect repellents containing diethyltoluamide; wearing long-sleeved shirts, long pants, and a hat when outdoors; and sleeping under an insecticide-treated bed net in an air-conditioned or a well-screened room are recommended. The prime times for mosquitoes to feed are at dawn and dusk, so taking caution and/or avoiding the outdoors during these times limits the hazard of exposure.[16–18]

Risks from Snake Bites

Displaced reptiles, such as snakes, are likely to be found after flooding and other natural disasters. It is advised to avoid snakes and leave them alone. Any attempt to kill snakes is both a danger and a risk. A disaster situation is dangerous enough without the added risk of a potentially venomous snakebite with limited resources for treatment.[18]

Leptospirosis Risk

Leptospirosis may occur in those who wade, swim, or bathe in waters contaminated by animal urine. The symptoms often mimic other acute febrile illnesses such as dengue and malaria, so HCPs should be mindful of patients presenting with headache, fever, chills, myalgia, nausea, diarrhea, abdominal pain, and occasionally a skin rash. Anyone working in floodwater should protect broken skin with a waterproof dressing and should ensure that they do not allow water to enter their mouth via the hands, food, or clothing. All food and drinking water should be protected to prevent contamination and drinking water boiled if in doubt because filtration does not prevent leptospirosis.[16–18,23]

Cleanup After a Disaster

Being aware of the preponderance of safety issues in the environment after a disaster has occurred is critical to the safety of HCPs. Buildings or structures that have not been examined by a certified inspector should be avoided and not entered until deemed safe. Appropriate clothing such as safety glasses, work gloves, waterproof boots, and hard hats should be worn for personal safety. All items that cannot be washed and disinfected should be removed and appropriately discarded. Carbon monoxide fumes from generators are extremely dangerous, and their use should be avoided or carefully monitored.[19,20]

PSYCHOLOGICAL AND EMOTIONAL CARE

Traumatic experiences from disasters can cause extreme stress because of the threat or experiences of loss of life and concerns regarding safety. During these events, there may be large loss of life, many serious injuries, missing and separated families or loved ones, and destruction of landscape as one remembers. These events cause ones' sense of security to be lost, thus causing feelings of helplessness and vulnerability. Common emotional reactions include feeling empty, sadness, anger, grief, anxiety, and irritability. Some individuals have difficulty functioning at home and work. Others report an inability to concentrate along with confusion, memory loss, and decision-making problems.

Physical reactions to disaster events may include symptoms such as fatigue, headaches, stomach aches, and aches and pains in general. Some may experience nightmares or recurring dreams about the disaster event. Whatever the case may be, it is extremely important for the HCP to recognize these symptoms and refer to appropriate mental health resources for counseling. Listening to the stories of the event may offer comfort on the road to recovery.[18,19]

Illness Abroad

HCPs and first responders are at risk for injury and illness when traveling into areas after a natural disaster. Therefore, identifying a doctor ahead of time as well as knowing medical resources that are available in the event of illness or injury are prudent actions. HCPs should be aware that available functioning hospitals or clinics may be overwhelmed treating victims of the disaster and unable to accommodate treatment of first responders. Consideration should be given to purchasing supplemental health insurance in the event that a serious illness requires evacuation out of or to other parts of the country to receive medical attention and care.[24]

Security

Americans traveling abroad should register with the American Embassy in the country of destination. During times of disaster, registration is extremely important because of disrupted communication services or remote locations. HCPs may be trying to help those affected by a disaster, but they also need to be aware that in some countries there may be restricted access to certain areas because of health or security concerns. Abiding by local laws helps to ensure safety.

First responders should keep passports and travel documents with them at all times, storing them in a waterproof bag. Family or friends should have copies of the HCP's passport and travel documents, an itinerary of travel plans, and contact information. It is also prudent to check in with family or friends at predetermined times.[24]

On Return Home

On return home from any disaster area, first responders who become ill for any reason should receive a medical evaluation. These evaluations should also include psychological support and counseling as necessary. Returning travelers should seek health care in the event of fever, rash, respiratory illness, or any other unusual symptoms. Illness including a fever or flulike symptoms either while traveling in a malaria-risk area or for up to 1 year after returning home should prompt immediate medical attention.[18,25]

SUMMARY

To prioritize the most common effects of a disaster, HCPs must decide in advance what is needed and how, when, and whom to provide the necessary support to deal with the posteffects of a disaster. During the rescue mission, the primary public health concern is clean drinking water, food, shelter, and medical care. Medical care is critical especially in areas where little or no medical care exists.

Natural disasters do not necessarily cause an increase in infectious disease outbreaks. However, contaminated water and food supplies as well as the lack of shelter and medical care may have a secondary effect of worsening illnesses that already exists in the affected region. Appropriate preparation in the form of preplanning for immunizations as well as education about other forms of protection, such as appropriate apparel and water decontamination, promotes a safer environment for first responders and survivors. The continued need for postdisaster health monitoring for HCPs is imperative.

The effects of a disaster last a long time; therefore there is an ongoing need to focus on the physical and environmental effects, including surveying and monitoring for infectious water or insect-transmitted diseases; restoring normal primary health services, water systems, transportation, housing, and employment; and continuing to assist the community's recovery after the immediate crisis has subsided.

REFERENCES

1. American Nurses Association (ANA). Adapting standards of care under extreme conditions: guidance for professionals during disasters, pandemics, and other extreme emergencies. ANA Center for Health Policy, Columbia University School of Nursing; 2008. Available at: http://www.nursingworld.org/HomepageCategory/NursingInsider/Archive_1/2008NI/Mar08NI/ANAIssuesPolicyPaperforHealthCareProfessionalsWhoRespondtoEmergenciesDisastersorPande.aspx. Accessed October 1, 2010.
2. Veenema TG, editor. Disaster nursing and emergency preparedness. 2nd edition. New York: Springer; 2007. p. 656.
3. Halpern P, Rosen B, Carasso S, et al. Intensive care in a field hospital in an urban disaster area: lessons from the 1999 earthquake in Turkey. Crit Care Med 2003; 31:1589–90.

4. Pan American Health Organization/World Health Organization. "Earthquake in Haiti: PAHO/WHO situation report on health activities post earthquake"; 2010. Available at: http://www.euro.who.int/en/what-we-do/health-topics/emergencies/disaster-preparedness-and-response/news2/news/2010/01/earthquake-devastat ion-in-hait. Accessed October 1, 2010.

5. Centers for Disease Control and Prevention Health Alert Network Notification, Clinician Outreach and Communication Activiry (COCA), CDC Emergency Communication System, CDC Health Advisory; 2010. Available at: http://emergency.cdc. gov/disasters/. Accessed October 1, 2010.

6. Campanella N. Infectious diseases and natural disasters: the effects of hurricane Mitch over Villanueva municipal area, Nicaragua. Public Health Rev 1999;27: 311–9.

7. Cockburn A, St Clair J, Silverstein K. The politics of natural disaster: who made hurricane Mitch so bad? Int J Health Serv 1999;29:459–62.

8. Wisner B, Adams J, editors. Environmental health in emergencies and disasters: a practical guide. Geneva (Switzerland): World Health Organization; 2002. p. 1998.

9. Harvey P, Baghri S, Reed B. Emergency sanitation: assessment and programme design. Leicestershire (UK): Water, Engineering and Development Centre, Loughborough University; 2002. Available at: http://www.who.int/water_sanitation_ health/hygiene/envsan/tn08/en/index.html. Accessed October 1, 2010.

10. Health in Emergencies and Disasters Pan American Health Organization (PAHO). 'Unseating the myths surrounding the management of cadavers', Disaster newsletter, No. 93, 2003. PAHO, USA. Geneva (Switzerland): WHO; 2003.

11. Oliver Morgan, Egbert Sondorp. Management of the dead following the South Asian tsunami disaster. 2005. Available at: http://www.omorgan.info/download/projects/Study%20Protocol%20%20Dead%20bodies%20after%20the%20Tsunami.pdf. Accessed June 27, 2010.

12. Morgan O. Infectious disease risk of dead bodies following natural disasters. Rev Panam Salud Publica 2004;15(5):307–12.

13. Pan American Health Organization. Management of dead bodies in disaster situations. Washington, DC: PAHO; 2004.

14. Centers for Disease Control and Prevention (CDC). Vaccinations. 2009. Available at: http://wwwnc.cdc.gov/travel/content/vaccinations.aspx. Accessed May 23, 2010.

15. Centers for Disease Control and Prevention (CDC). Infectious disease information. 2007. Available at: http://www.cdc.gov/ncidod/diseases/submenus/sub_ cholera.htm. Accessed May 23, 2010.

16. Centers for Disease Control and Prevention (CDC). Chapter 2 The pre-travel consultation travel-related vaccine-preventable diseases. 2007. Available at: http://wwwnc. cdc.gov/travel/yellowbook/2010/chapter-2/yellow-fever.aspx. Accessed July 9, 2010.

17. Centers for Disease Control and Prevention (CDC). Malaria. Available at: http://www.cdc.gov/MALARIA. Accessed June 16, 2010.

18. Centers for Disease Control and Prevention (CDC). Health recommendations for relief workers responding to disasters. 2010. Available at: http://wwwnc.cdc.gov/travel/content/relief-workers.aspx. Accessed June 16, 2010.

19. American Red Cross. Preparedness fast facts: Emergency-specific preparedness information. 2010. Available at: http://wwwnc.cdc.gov/travel/content/relief-workers.aspx. Accessed July 10, 2010.

20. Centers for Disease Control and Prevention (CDC). Available at: http://wwwnc.cdc. gov/travel/yellowbook/2010/chapter-2/water-disinfection.aspx. Accessed July 7, 2010.
21. Backer HD. Field water disinfection. In: Auerbach PS, editor. Wilderness medicine. 5th edition. Philadelphia: Mosby; 2007. p. 1368–417.
22. Hamilton MG, Lundy PM. Medical countermeasures to WMDs: defense research for civilian and military use. Toxicology 2007;233(1-3):8–12.
23. The Leptospirosis Information Center. Available at: http://www.leptospirosis.org/ topic.php?t=24. Accessed July 8, 2010.
24. U.S. Department of State. Available at: http://travel.state.gov/travel/tips/tips_ 1232.html. Accessed July 10, 2010.
25. American Red Cross. Be Red Cross ready. Returning home after a hurricane or flood. 2009. Available at: http://www.tallyredcross.org/py_tsunamis.html. Accessed July 7, 2010.

Cultural, Ethical, and Spiritual Competencies of Health Care Providers Responding to a Catastrophic Event

Mini M. Jose, PhD, RN

KEYWORDS

- Culture • Spirituality • Ethics • Disaster • Competency
- Provider

Health care providers responding to catastrophic events are under tremendous pressure as they deal with the complex physical, psychological, cultural, spiritual, and ethical dimensions of the care they provide to disaster victims. They are expected to display cultural sensitivity when they may be unaware of the cultural norms and practices of the disaster-stricken population. They are also expected to take care of victims' spiritual distress when their own soul may be suffering. Cultural and spiritual practices and beliefs may vary widely among individuals even within the same culture, and therefore the difficulty in prudently providing culturally competent, ethically sound, and spiritually appropriate care to disaster victims is understandable.

Practicing within the framework of an ethic of care is an expectation of health care providers; however, the difficulties associated with upholding values associated with the ethic of care are exacerbated during a disaster. As at all other times, health care providers are expected to adhere to ethical principles outlined in their codes of ethics and legal parameters that delineate their professional practice. Unfortunately, during a disaster these guidelines may provide no clear directives because roles, relationships, settings, equipment, and the patient population itself become varied and sometimes unpredictable, challenging decision-making abilities.[1–4] For example, in situations involving communicable diseases in which quarantine is enforced, health care providers may have to restrict victims' right to autonomy, freedom of movement, lifestyle, and access to personal property. Fair allocation of scarce resources, such as food, shelter, and health care services, to the "most needy among the equally needy" is another example of ethical decision making health care providers face. Triaging

---

The author has nothing to disclose.

School of Nursing, University of Texas Medical Branch, Mail Route 1029, Galveston, TX 77555, USA

E-mail address: mmjose@utmb.edu

victims at a disaster site, which may result in some receiving care while others die, is an ethical dilemma health care providers face as they are forced to weigh between the principles of beneficence (doing good) and nonmaleficence (doing no harm).

During a disaster, health care providers need to function with integrity and sensitivity; therefore, it is critical that clear guidelines be developed and resources provided to enhance the cultural, ethical, and spiritual competencies of health care providers who respond to the call of duty.

CULTURAL COMPETENCE

The United Nations Educational, Scientific, and Cultural Organization (UNESCO) declared that culture takes diverse forms across time and space.[5] This diversity is embodied in the uniqueness and plurality of the identities of the groups and societies making up humankind. UNESCO's universal declaration on cultural diversity holds that as a source of exchange, innovation, and creativity, cultural diversity is as necessary for humankind as biodiversity is for nature, and therefore it is imperative that health care providers understand the cultural diversity and cultural practices of a given society to provide culturally sensitive care to them. Nazarchuk and Legg[6] caution that the ideal of cultural competence should not be disregarded during disasters because doing so violates professional integrity and health care providers' commitment to provide holistic care to individuals, families, and communities.

Health care providers are expected to answer the call of duty at disaster sites—locally, regionally, nationally, and internationally. The complexity of providing culturally sensitive care generally increases as the geographic distance to the location of the disaster increases, largely because of health care providers' unfamiliarity with the cultural practices and norms of the people living in and around the site of disaster. Cornelison[7] identifies autonomy clashes between patients and health professionals, including end-of-life values and preferences, cultural responses to pain, pain management, and the problem of stereotypical and uncaring behaviors toward people different from them as the major issues that can affect provider and patient interactions during a disaster.

When dealing with diverse cultures, health care providers must avoid the traps of cultural stereotypy and ethnocentrism. Many health-related cultural practices, such as rituals associated with birth and death, dietary practices, and ways of living unique to the disaster-stricken population, can have a profound impact on physical and psychological well-being and recovery. Cultural sensitivity should be emphasized in the disaster-preparedness curriculum of all health care providers, and to that end they should be given information about available resources. A working knowledge of the culture and language at the geographic region of disaster ensures accurate communication between health care providers and victims.

Cultural sensitivity should be maintained in the provision of care and in the selection and distribution of resources to the victims. The cultural competency of health care providers is a key element in establishing trust and credibility within a community suffering from human and material loss in the aftermath of a disaster. Yang and colleagues[2] found that if the disaster-stricken area comprises ethnic groups with different cultures, traditions, and languages, obtaining local help becomes very difficult because of the inability to communicate. The provision of humanitarian aid and health care becomes much more complex when providers are responding to a disaster in a foreign country.

Amarasiri de Silva[8] studied disaster response during the December 2004 tsunami in Sri Lanka and pointed out that ignoring local networks during humanitarian aid by international agencies to speed up recovery may in fact have led to a flare up of ethnic tensions and unfair treatment of poor segments of society. It is recommended that health care providers be sensitive to ethnic sentiments and that local networks are rightly consulted to increase social harmony and ethnic neutrality in a disaster-hit, multiethnic population. Local networks provide an easily accessible asset regarding the cultural practices of disaster-hit communities.

Cultural rituals and practices dominate the lives of people in many ways, especially through celebrating cultural heritage in their life events, such as birth, death, marriage, and attaining maturity. During a disaster, when corpses are disposed of at the earliest opportunity to prevent public health hazards, families who are unable to complete death rituals of their loved ones should be given psychological support to prevent dysfunctional grieving, which could precipitate mental anguish or illnesses.

Andrulis and colleagues[9] contend that one lesson learned from a national-level disaster, such as Hurricane Katrina, is the need to focus on diversity during disaster preparedness, because cooperation from all racial and ethnic populations is required during disaster response. The lessons learned from these disasters indicate the direction that future preparedness efforts must take to fully integrate factors related to race, culture, and language into risk communication, public health training, measurement, coordination, and policy at all levels. Planning and preparation are vital to the success of disaster relief operations and involve the commitment of each provider to seek out and effectively use available resources.

Health care providers must be nonjudgmental and respectful to each individual to establish a trusting relationship. If a language barrier is a hindrance, providers must use the services of translators or automated translation services. Books and the Internet can help providers acquire knowledge about the cultural practices, social norms, and ways of living so that they are able to select and provide culturally appropriate resources, such as clothing, food, and other basic necessities for all age groups. Cultural sensitivity becomes a daunting task in a multicultural and multilingual society. Leininger's[10] transcultural nursing theory is a useful framework for health care professionals to use in understanding cultural dimensions during health and illness. Leininger defined transcultural nursing as a humanistic and scientific area of formal study and practice in nursing, focused on differences and similarities among cultures, that is based on cultural values, beliefs, and practices. He postulated that to provide care, nurses must understand and appreciate inherent differences and similarities not only locally but also regionally, nationally, and worldwide.

Cultural and religious preferences should be considered when making decisions about victims' treatment regimens. If cultural norms are challenged during the provision of care, however technically and scientifically superior the care, it will not provide the intended comfort to the victim and may be perceived as demeaning and result in demoralization of the affected society.

Giger and Davidhizar's[11] transcultural assessment model provides a framework for patient assessment and from which culturally sensitive care can be designed. The model includes six cultural phenomena, including (1) communication, (2) time, (3) space, (4) social organization, (5) environmental control, and (6) biologic variations. Providers must familiarize themselves with institutional policies and guidelines from health and welfare agencies, such as the Centers for Disease Control and Prevention (CDC), the World Health Organization (WHO), and the International Federation of Red Cross and Red Crescent societies (IFRC).[12–14] Tuhkanen and George[15] suggest that community participation involving disaster-affected people and the local community, especially women, in health development projects helps ensure both success and sustainability.

ETHICAL COMPETENCE

The ethical implications of health care providers' response to a disaster begins with the decision to respond to a disaster event, because this always involves the danger of putting one's own life on the line. Barr and colleagues,[16] who studied the ethical decision-making process of health care workers during a natural disaster, found that one-third of the health care workforce may not be available to respond to a pandemic disaster because of perceived risk to their own health, the need to care for their own children at home, and a projected 15% of the health care workforce already affected by the disaster.

DeSimone[17] reported that employees are less likely to report to duty if the cause of disaster is biologic or chemical in nature, with an unknown origin. Of course, this situation might create another ethical dilemma for the health care administrator who must organize care with an understaffed and overstretched workforce, increasing the health risks to those who respond to the duty to care. The American Medical Association (AMA) code of ethics upholds that "when participating in disaster responses, physicians should balance immediate benefits to the individual patients with the ability to care for patients in the future."[18] The American Nurses Association (ANA) code of ethics Provision 3 states "the nurse promotes, advocates for and strives to protect the health, safety, and rights of the patient," whereas Provision 5 of the code states "the nurse owes the same duties to self as to others, including the responsibility to preserve integrity and safety."[19] Essentially, professional codes of ethics require health care providers to balance risk and benefit between their own safety and their duty to care.

During a disaster, ethical codes can be ambiguous and do not always provide clear directives, allowing freedom for interpretation and personal choice by health care providers.[19,20] Malm and colleagues[21] examined the ethics of disaster to clear this ambiguity and found that the duty to treat is grounded on five factors: (1) the health care provider's consent given at the time of signing the employment contract, (2) implied consent to treat patients through choosing a health care career, (3) special training received to perform the duty, (4) reciprocity or the social contract implied through the subsidization of health care education with an expectation that the health care professional will serve the society in times of need, and (5) the professional oaths and codes that are binding to professional responsibilities. The authors further suggest that to avoid absenteeism during an emergency, it is beneficial to create a corps of workers who sign an expressed consent with associated perks to be bound to respond to a disaster. The authors also hailed the hurricane preparedness plan developed by the city of Galveston in Texas as a disaster-preparedness model that could be adopted nationwide.

The universal principles of bioethics involve autonomy (right to choose and consent), beneficence (doing good), nonmaleficence (doing no harm), and justice (distributive fairness). Triage is the well-established process of finding the most appropriate disposition for a patient based on an assessment of the patient's illness and its urgency. Wynia[22] identified the "three R's" of health care disasters and public health emergencies:

1. Rationing of vaccines, medications, food, and other consumables depending on the triage decisions.
2. Restrictions on people's liberties/access to and from health care services and from their personal resources, especially during a pandemic or biologic weapon attacks when isolation and quarantine are enforced.
3. Responsibilities of health care professionals to continue providing care and treatment, even when doing so places them, their families, and others close to them at risk.

During disasters, health care providers are required to assume roles and responsibilities for which they were not specialized, that are both in and out of their comfort zone, and often must deviate from the standards and practices they are accustomed to in their regular roles. Yang and colleagues[2] reported on the real-time ethical dilemmas encountered by Chinese nurses who participated in the Wenchuan earthquake disaster response that occurred in May 2008. When they had to work without an adequate supply of equipment and consumables, these nurses creatively used mineral water to clean surgical instruments, iodine to disinfect, and converted intravenous tubing into urinary catheters. Although these nurses questioned themselves about the correctness of their interventions, saving the lives of victims underpinned their actions. These nurses rose above their comfort zones to adapt their standards to the disaster situation; in fact, they reported doing the work of cooks, janitors, teachers, and engineers.

Allocation of scarce resources to the "most needy among the equally needy" is a challenging ethical dilemma for health care providers responding to disasters. Triage decisions can easily become discriminatory. For example, if there is an order to triage based on age, sex, race, or any type of vulnerability other than accepted utilitarian principles, the triage process becomes a discriminatory practice, and prudent health care providers should question the decision-making process.

Eisenman and colleagues[23] caution that people with chronic medical and mental illness or disability are at particular risk during disasters and are less likely to have enough supplies during a disaster. Barr and colleagues[16] suggest that several contrasting techniques may be considered to rationalize care, such as using a quality-adjusted life-year's technique that gives priority to younger individuals or triage techniques based on a utilitarian approach, which delivers the greatest medical benefit to the greatest number of people.

Responding to the recent earthquake in Haiti, Merin and colleagues[1] used a simple algorithm consisting of three questions to ensure a fair triaging process:

1. How urgent is this patient's condition?
2. Do we have adequate resources to meet this patient's needs?
3. Assuming we admit this patient and provide the level of care required, can the patient's life be saved?

They also created an ad hoc ethics committee in which the attending physician presented the case to a panel of three senior physicians before a treatment decision was made. The author also highlighted the benefit of early discharge, stating that most patients were discharged the very next day, thus allowing a hospital with a 75-bed capacity to attend to 100 patients a day. Although the cornerstone of managing rising surge capacity is to provide care for a greater number of people, early discharge raises serious questions about quality of care. Krauss and colleagues[24] discussed the issue of inpatient surge capacity and stated that during overwhelming disasters, health systems must be considered lifeboats with insufficient capacity to minister to all. Thus, decisions regarding who is best served by the lifeboat must be made based on the guiding principles of medical ethics, utilitarian perspectives, expected clinical benefits, and the principle of proportionality in which the needs of all, including those "in the boat" and those "still in the water," are considered on equal terms.

Triage is the most accepted method of allocating scarce resources, and usually follows the egalitarian ethical principle that focuses on the needs of individuals. During a disaster, a shift in the ethics of triage to a utilitarian perspective focused on the needs of the community is warranted, and Tabery and Mackett[25] argue that triage review boards at the local, regional, and national level should collectively decide when the move from egalitarian to utilitarian triage be made. Occasionally, general guidelines of triage may be challenged and special considerations must be made when the affected population involves dignitaries, prisoners, or criminals. Health care providers must examine and control their own biases to ensure fair and just allocation of scarce resources.

Another issue with ethical implications is the restriction or violation of patient's rights that are invariably respected in normal circumstances. Informed consent might not be possible in all circumstances of treatment and research. Pearlman[26] suggests that each state health department should establish an Institutional Review Board (IRB) to ensure oversight of ethical research and provide expedited review during disaster research. Another area of possible violation of patients' autonomy involves the imposition of restrictions, such as quarantine or restricting access to family and property. Individual choices should be examined in light of the greatest good for the rest of the society. Restrictions should be explained in a calm and reassuring manner so that the victims can be participants in the disaster response process. Clear, concise, and empathetic communication from the health care provider can help alleviate anxieties and misgivings of the victims and the community. Protecting the privacy and confidentiality of patient information is another ethical challenge when media attention is focused on disaster victims.

SPIRITUAL COMPETENCE

Given that spirituality is an important dimension of holistic health, the healing process is not complete without spiritual care. Gunn[27] stated that when a tragedy occurs, whether through profound personal loss or the global impact of a community, regional, or national disaster, it can strike at the very heart of humankind's view of self and the world, and, for believers, understanding of God's role in human events.

Spirituality involves relationships with things beyond the physical and material world, including a Supreme Being or higher power. The nursing profession deems spirituality as an integral part of holistic nursing and believes that every individual has spiritual needs of some kind. Spiritual care is often considered a complementary or alternative therapy intervention. A person's spirituality is greatly challenged in times of disaster and it is important to provide attention to spiritual needs along with the physical needs of victims. Silent spiritual suffering and the confusion that victims are experiencing are often ignored in the chaos of a disaster. Similarly, the overwhelming physical and psychological demands of caregiving and the enormous losses witnessed also may challenge the spirituality of health care providers, and it is critical that responders do not lose sight of their own spiritual needs.

Often spirituality is equated with religion and it is very important for health care providers to understand the distinction between religion and spirituality. Religiosity includes subscribing to certain beliefs, forms of worship, practices, and cultural identity. Spirituality conveys a voyage of self-actualization toward oneness with the universe. Unfortunately, the humanitarian aid efforts by faith-based nongovernmental organizations are often tainted by the hidden motives of proselytizing work or religious conversion, and this can create religious doubts and be spiritually distressing for disaster victims.[28] Health care workers should not encourage these activities by faith-based organizations, because they violate victim autonomy and exploit the vulnerability of the community.

During a study conducted among the tsunami-hit population in India, Rajkumar and colleagues[29] asked the victims to identify the most important coping mechanism they used for their survival, finding that most participants claimed religious beliefs as the most important factor contributing to their survival. The authors further argue that religious beliefs and rituals create a social and collective existence, minimizing the feelings of loss and isolation in a disaster-hit community, and that intervention after disaster should be grounded in ethnocultural beliefs and practices.

A research study conducted by Hanson and colleagues[30] found that spiritual care activities are varied and that health care providers are increasingly asked to assume responsibility for spiritual care, but that their willingness and ability to do so is debated. This study affirms that spiritual preparation and response by health care providers is imperative in a disaster situation, especially when clergy and other spiritual resources are not immediately available.

Carpenter[31] suggests that nurses engage in spiritual care for patients by following some essential steps: (1) evaluating and reflecting on their own sense of spirituality, (2) finding ways to nurture their own spirituality, (3) acknowledging purpose and meaning of their work, and (4) entering each patient relationship with intentionality or a clear mind to focus on the patient assigned to their care. Responding to a disaster is taxing physically and psychologically, and providers must identify and work through their emotions while preparing themselves spiritually. Health care providers with broken spirits will not be able to heal the physiologic or psychological wounds of grieving individuals or a disaster-stricken community.

RESOURCES FOR HEALTH CARE PROVIDERS

The history of humankind shows that natural and human-made disasters can occur at any time, and preparedness is key to the successful resolution of a disastrous event. Fortunately a heightened awareness is evident in the health care community through disaster preparedness. Often major catastrophic events involving thousands of lost lives attract global attention and international agencies, and foreign governments extend helping hands to the disaster-stricken population.

Humanitarian aid efforts and resources from international agencies are highly valuable for providing health care in a disaster area, and specialized training and protocols available from international agencies should be welcomed and integrated with the efforts of the local agencies. The International Red Cross Society (IRCS), the WHO, and the Nursing Emergency Preparedness Education Coalition (NEPEC) have many resources to help registered nurses acquire knowledge and skills regarding disaster preparedness.[32–34]

While providing care during the Haitian earthquake, Roseborough[35] observed that health care providers with specialized training in disaster relief provided much better care with fewer resources and were in line with international standards and guidelines compared with another team that adopted a warzone approach in which human dignity and standards of care were often overlooked. Unlike the United States–based disaster response grounded on the Incident Command System structure, international disaster response is coordinated by the United Nations Office for Coordination of Humanitarian Affairs (OCHA) through its "cluster" system. Each cluster (eg, health, food, shelter, water, sanitation) is headed by a separate OCHA agency, and these clusters communicate with each other, constantly focusing on performance improvement. The sphere project is a collaboration of major international aid organizations that has established international standards for shelter, food, water, sanitation, and protection. Health care providers must be familiar with the sphere project and OCHA cluster systems, either through online resources or short courses offered by international agencies, so that humane and responsible care is provided during a disaster-relief operation.

Another document that guides humanitarian decision making and coordination is the "code of conduct for the International Red Cross and Red Crescent Movement and Non-Governmental Organizations (NGOs) in Disaster Relief" drafted and launched just after the Rwanda genocide of April 1994.[36] Health care providers who are familiar with the 10 articles of this document are prepared to provide competent care without losing sight of ethical, moral, cultural, and spiritual aspects of human beings in need of care during a catastrophic event.

Nationally and locally most governmental and nongovernmental institutions have their own disaster management plans, and health care providers are expected to function within the framework of the institutional policies. To ensure the competency of health care providers, the Joint Commission mandates that every health care organization engage in disaster preparedness planning, regularly conducting drills that incorporate evidence-based practices.[37,38] Clear guidelines are still lacking in many areas of disaster preparedness, and providers often must operate with limited resources. In addition to referencing professional literature, health care providers must also use guidelines from humanitarian aid agencies because these organizations focus on compassionate aid, ensuring recognition of and respect for cultural diversity, human dignity, and justice to the affected population.

SUMMARY

Compassion is a language that is understood across cultures, religions, and nations. Being compassionate and empathetic is a basic responsibility of health care providers responding to disasters. Compassion and empathy cannot be operationalized unless providers show culturally competent, ethically right, and spiritually caring behavior. In addition to being accepting of cultures other than their own, providers must read literature and familiarize themselves with the predominant cultures of the affected population. Ethically right decision making is essentially an act of balancing the risks and benefits to the entire society.

Spiritual care is an important dimension of total health, and therefore recognition and resolution of the spiritual needs of disaster victims is an essential role of health care providers. Disaster management is teamwork and therefore requires that health care providers draw on the expertise and support of other team members; coordinating efforts with local religious, social governmental organizations, and NGOs to deal with the intangible effects of the cultural and spiritual impact of a disaster and to prevent further demoralization of the affected community is imperative. Disasters occur, and the only thing that can ameliorate their devastating effects is to improve disaster preparedness and respond collectively and courageously to every catastrophic event.

REFERENCES

1. Merin O, Ash N, Levy G, et al. The Israeli field hospital in Haiti—ethical dilemmas in early disaster response. N Engl J Med 2010;362(11):e38.
2. Yang Y, Xiao L, Cheng H, et al. Chinese nurses' experience in the Wenchuan earthquake relief. Int Nurs Rev 2010;57:217–23.
3. Johnstone M. Health care disaster ethics: a call to action. Aust Nurs J 2009; 17:27.
4. Holt R. Making difficult ethical decisions in patient care during natural disasters and other mass casualty events. Otolaryngol Head Neck Surg 2008; 139:181–6.

5. Unesco. Universal declaration on cultural diversity. Available at: http://unesdoc. unesco.org/images/0012/001271/127160m.pdf. Accessed May 20, 2010.
6. Nazarchuk SA, Legg TJ. Cultural considerations in a disaster. In: Adelman DS, Legg TJ, editors. Disaster nursing: a handbook for practice. Sudbury (MA): Jones and Bartlett; 2008. p. 75–84.
7. Cornelison A. Cultural barriers to compassionate care—patients' and health professionals' perspectives. Bioethics Forum 2001;17(1):7–14.
8. Amarasiri de Silva MW. Ethnicity, politics and inequality: post tsunami humanitarian aid delivery in Ampara District, Sri Lanka. Disasters 2009;33:253–73.
9. Andrulis D, Siddiqui N, Gantner J. Preparing racially and ethnically diverse communities for public health emergencies. Health Aff 2007;26:1269–79.
10. Leininger M. Transcultural nursing: the study and practice field. Imprint 1991;38: 55–66.
11. Giger J, Davidhizar R. The Giger and Davidhizar transcultural assessment model. J Transcult Nurs 2002;13:185–8.
12. Center of Disease Control (CDC). The risk communicator. Available at: http://emergency.cdc.gov/ercn/02/index.asp. Accessed August 9, 2010.
13. World Health Organization (WHO). Managing WHO humanitarian response in the field. Available at: http://www.wpro.who.int/NR/rdonlyres/FDDE6DC7-09D6-4BE9-9DC1-4D3D058B8DE9/0/managing_who_humanitarian_response_in_the_field_25june2008.pdf. Accessed August 10, 2010.
14. International Federation of Red Cross and Red Crescent Societies (IFRC). Ethics in disaster response. Available at: http://www.ifrc.org/what/disasters/responding/ethics.asp. Accessed August 10, 2010.
15. Tuhkanen S, George K. A disaster preparedness and response project in Afghanistan: participants' perceptions. J Adv Nurs 2008;64:287–97.
16. Barr H, Macfarlane J, Macgregor O, et al. Ethical planning for an influenza pandemic. Clin Med 2008;8:49–52.
17. DeSimone C. Response of public health workers to various emergencies. AAOHN J 2009;57:17–23.
18. American Medical Association. Physician obligation in disaster preparedness and response. Available at: http://www.ama-assn.org/ama/pub/physician-resources/medical-ethics/code-medical-ethics/opinion9067.shtml. Accessed August 10, 2010.
19. American Nurses Association. Code of ethics for nurses with interpretive statements. Washington, DC: American Nurses Publishing; 2001. p. 5–7.
20. Grimaldi M. Ethical decisions in times of disaster: choices healthcare workers must make. J Trauma Nurs 2007;14:163–4.
21. Malm H, May T, Francis L, et al. Ethics, pandemics, and the duty to treat. Am J Bioeth 2008;8:4–19.
22. Wynia M. Ethics and public health emergencies: encouraging responsibility. Am J Bioeth 2007;74:1–4.
23. Eisenman D, Zhou Q, Ong M, et al. Variations in disaster preparedness by mental health, perceived general health, and disability status. Disaster Med Public Health Prepared 2009;3:33–41.
24. Kraus C, Levy F, Kelen G. Lifeboat ethics: considerations in the discharge of inpatients for the creation of hospital surge capacity. Disaster Med Public Health Prepared 2007;1:51–6.
25. Tabery J, Mackett C, University of Pittsburgh Medical Center Pandemic Influenza Task Force's Triage Review Board. Ethics of triage in the event of an Influenza pandemic. Disaster Med Public Health Prepared 2008;2:114–8.

26. Perlman D. Public health practice vs. research: implications for preparedness and disaster research review by state health department IRBs. Disaster Med Public Health Prepared 2008;2:185–91.
27. Gunn F. Spiritual issues in the aftermath of disaster. Southampt Med J 2007;100: 936–7.
28. Jayasinghe S. Faith-based NGOs and healthcare in poor countries: a preliminary exploration of ethical issues. Med Ethics 2007;33:623–6.
29. Rajkumar A, Premkumar T, Tharyan P. Coping with the Asian tsunami: perspectives from Tamil Nadu, India on the determinants of resilience in the face of adversity. Soc Sci Med 2008;67:844–53.
30. Hanson L, Dobbs D, Usher B, et al. Providers and types of spiritual care during serious illness. J Palliat Med 2008;11:907–14.
31. Carpenter K, Girvin L, Kitner W, et al. Spirituality: dimensions in critical care nursing. Dimens Crit Care Nurs 2008;271:16–20.
32. International Committee of the Red Cross (ICRC). Humanitarian assistance training H.E.L.P. I (Health Emergencies in Large Populations) H.E.L.P. II (Health, Ethics, Law and Policies). Available at: http://www.icrc.org/Web/eng/siteeng0.nsf/html/help_course?OpenDocument. Accessed August 11, 2010.
33. World Health organization (WHO). Health cluster guide. Available at: http://www.who.int/hac/global_health_cluster/guide/en/index.html. Accessed August 8, 2010.
34. Nursing Emergency Preparedness Education Coalition (NEPEC). Nursing curriculum plan for emergency preparedness. Available at: http://www.nursing.vanderbilt.edu/incmce/curriculum.html. Accessed August 11, 2010.
35. Roseborough S. A tale of two responses: Haiti earthquake highlights the need for training in international disaster response. Disaster Med Public Health Prepared 2010;4:21–3.
36. Hilhorst D. Dead letter or living document? Ten years of the code of conduct for disaster relief. Disasters 2005;29:351–69.
37. The Joint Commission. Emergency preparedness. Available at: http://www.jointcommission.org/NR/rdonlyres/9C8DE572-5D7A-4F28-AB84-3741EC82AF98/0/emergencypreparedness.pdf. Accessed August 10, 2010.
38. Joint Commission on Accreditation of Healthcare Organizations. Surge hospitals: providing safe care in emergencies. Available at: http://www.jointcommission.org/NR/rdonlyres/802E9DA4-AE80-4584-A205-48989C5BD684/0/surgehospital.pdf. Accessed August 7, 2010.

Keeping PEDIATRICS in Pediatric Disaster Management: Before, During, and in the Aftermath of Complex Emergencies

Frances Kelly, MSN, RN

KEYWORDS

- Disaster management • Complex emergency • Children
- Emergency pediatrics

Historically, whether naturally occurring or human-made, there has been no dearth of disasters. From 1900 until the turn of the twenty-first century, there have been more than 9800 natural disasters[1] affecting more than 67 million children worldwide.[2] The number of disasters is expected to increase significantly over the next several years, as a result of population growth, war, an increase in weather-related events,[3,4] changes in the global economy, and an increase in infections[3] especially due to terrorism.[5]

Although there is no discrimination in either the types of disasters or the region of the world in which they occur, children, the financially disadvantaged, mentally ill and physically disabled persons, as well as many women, racial minorities, and the elderly suffer a disproportionately high disaster risk compared with that of the general population.[6–8] Because of unique physical, developmental, and psychosocial characteristics of children, caring for them during complex emergencies is different than caring for adults.[9] However, planning for these unique physical, developmental, and psychosocial needs has not been well addressed when planning for complex emergencies.[10,11] Therefore, the purpose of this article is to review those characteristics of children that place them at higher disaster risk, and discuss the preparations necessary to meet their needs before, during, and in the aftermath of complex emergencies.

Ben Taub General Hospital, Harris County Hospital District, 1504 Taub Loop, Houston, TX 77030, USA
E-mail address: Frances_kelly@hchd.tmc.edu

Crit Care Nurs Clin N Am 22 (2010) 465–480
doi:10.1016/j.ccell.2010.10.005   ccnursing.theclinics.com
0899-5885/10/$ – see front matter © 2010 Elsevier Inc. All rights reserved.

SCOPE OF THE PROBLEM

Disasters or complex emergencies can result from naturally occurring phenomena or from human-made events. Several definitions of disaster, crisis, and emergency exist in the literature. According to the World Health Organization (1992),[12] a disaster can be ecological and psychosocial, and results in severe disruption which exceeds a community's ability to cope. McFarlane and Norris[13] defined disaster as a "potentially traumatic event that is collectively experienced, has an acute onset, and is time-delimited." A complex emergency exists during times of war, when people may be displaced from their homes, or when food is scarce or procuring it is risky, resulting in poor nutrition and an increased risk of mortality.[14]

Cicero and Baum[15] defined disasters as incidents or events of such a size that available resources are overwhelmed. Markovitz[16] defined disaster as any event that is unpredictable in nature, scope, and impact. Crisis, emergency, or disaster is described by Turner and colleagues[17] as any situation resulting from natural events such as earthquakes, famines, or floods, or from human-made events such as war. For the purposes of this article, the terms disaster and complex emergency will be used interchangeably, and will refer to any situation, whether naturally occurring or human-made, which substantially increases the need for and use of pediatric resources, and has the potential to overwhelm a hospital, a system, or a geographic region.

Children Are Not Small Adults

Children have unique physical, developmental, and psychosocial characteristics[18–22] that increase their risk of morbidity and mortality during disasters. Children are physically smaller and have immature or underdeveloped motor skills and abilities,[10,19,20,23] which may reduce the ability to perform self-care or impede escape. Children have a higher body surface area to mass ratio,[20] which predisposes them to hypothermia. Children generally have a thinner epidermis, which increases the risk of dehydration, exposure, and absorption of more chemical, biologic, radiological, and nuclear (CBRN) agents per kilogram.[10,20,23,24] In addition, children have a faster respiratory rate, thus increasing the potential to inhale more airborne pathogens than adults[10,20,23,24]; they also have a smaller amount of circulating blood volume, predisposing them to hypovolemia and shock.[20]

Children are developmentally immature and psychologically vulnerable.[19,20,25–28] This developmental immaturity influences a child's reaction to a disaster,[29] and significantly reduces their ability to accurately and quickly assess situational risk, increasing their risk of falling prey to those who wish to exploit them for sex, rape, prostitution, or to engage in human trafficking, to name but a few examples.[30–32] Evidence suggests that children may be more vulnerable if they are directly exposed to a disaster, suffer an injury or witness death, if they experience loss or grief, ongoing stress related to displacement or evacuation, or the loss of comforting surroundings, routines, and friends.[33]

Children are particularly vulnerable during complex emergencies, and are more likely to become victims or die.[10,22,30,34–40] A greater number of children live in poverty[30] (US Census Bureau, 2009) or overcrowded conditions as compared with those in the general population, further increasing their risk during disasters of contracting tuberculosis, measles, or human immunodeficiency virus.[14,30] Children suffering the highest risk of morbidity and mortality are those younger than 5 years who have been either abandoned or orphaned,[41] or who are living among a displaced population.[42] Conditions frequently cited as the cause of death in these children are very similar to those conditions that exist for many children around the world, even during nonemergency conditions, and include diarrhea, malnutrition, malaria, measles, and respiratory infections.[14,30,42–44]

During 1991, 63% of all the children younger than 5 years died among the Kurdish refugees along the Turkey-Iraq border.[44,45] In 1992, 74% of the children younger than 5 died during the famine in Somalia.[46] More than half of the children younger than 5 years died among the Rwandan and Burundian refugees in the Democratic Republic of the Congo in 1996.[47] Neonatal and maternal deaths were approximately 16% of all reported deaths among the Burundian refugees in the United Republic of Tanzania in 1998.[48] Neonatal deaths accounted for approximately 19% of all deaths among Afghan refugees in Pakistan.[49]

Pediatric and neonatal deaths during complex emergencies are not limited to those occurring in developing countries. Eighteen children and one 19-year-old were killed in the Oklahoma City bombing.[50] A total of 15 children were killed, including the 2 gunmen, during the Columbine High School shootings.[51] More than 3000 children lost a parent during the attack on September 11, 2001 in New York City.[52] And of the estimated 5.8 million people who lived in the areas hardest hit by Hurricane Katrina, more than 1 million lived in poverty,[53] and well over 1 million were likely children. The impact to children during complex emergencies, especially those resulting from terrorism, can be severe.[5] There are numerous CBRN agents that children may be exposed to in both deliberate and accidental events.[10,54,55]

Health Care Systems, Community Systems, and Providers Ill Prepared for Disasters Involving Children

Children comprise approximately 27.5% of the total United States population as of 2009.[56] Despite children comprising more than one-quarter of the total United States population, health care and community systems remain generally unprepared to effectively or efficiently address the physical, developmental, or psychological needs of children in a complex emergency.[38,57] Many local and regional areas have limited pediatric beds and pediatric competencies, which may negatively affect or reduce surge capacity.[57] There is an estimated 250 hospitals dedicated solely to the care of children,[58] representing a paltry 2% of the total number of registered and community hospitals in the United States.[59] There is clearly a disparity between the proportion of children in the United States population and the proportion of hospital beds dedicated to the care of children during stable conditions or during complex emergencies.[60] Seasonal variation in pediatric bed occupancy may further reduce the availability of pediatric beds during an emergency.[60]

There is a paucity of evidence available by which to determine the appropriate number of hospital beds needed for a surge in pediatric capacity.[60] The results of a simulation study conducted using New York City as the hypothetical setting revealed that under normal conditions, nearby hospitals could reliably accommodate approximately 250 patients per million population,[60] only half of the target surge capacity.[61] Accurately predicting pediatric surge resulting from a bioterrorism or pandemic event is difficult,[62] and evidence suggests that current pediatric resources will often fall short of meeting the needs of children in a large-scale event.[63]

Results of a survey returned by 1932 prehospital emergency medical services agencies indicated that less than half of the participating agencies included any pediatric simulation scenarios in disaster drills. Although a majority of the agencies did have written disaster plans, only 13.3% of them had plans for the pediatric patients, only 19.2% indicated the use of a pediatric specific triage protocol, and only 12.3% included pediatricians in planning. Most agencies did not include any disaster or emergency planning for a school-related event or for children with disabilities or special needs,[64] nor did they include pediatricians in planning for complex emergencies.[22,35] Consistent with this evidence, while it is known that children are most vulnerable during disasters or complex emergencies, not enough pediatric-specific equipment is kept on ambulances,[65,66] there are no standard pediatric-specific triage protocols in use during the prehospital phase of a complex emergency,[64] and children younger than 5 years receive fewer prehospital interventions than those older than 5 years.[67]

Despite a clear and compelling need for evidence-based, age-appropriate guidelines for the care of children in disasters and complex emergencies,[14,57] they do not exist in a single-source, comprehensive form.[14,17] An extensive search of the literature conducted by Turner and colleagues[17] revealed only 6 pediatric guidelines that included health care interventions for child and perinatal health in disasters. None of the 6 guidelines found were based on a systematic review of the literature or included recommendations linked to research supporting their inclusion. Moreover, although most school districts do have emergency management plans, there is wide variation among them according to the United States Government Accountability Office.[68]

Many of the pediatric care guidelines that do exist are written for use by physicians[69] and are intended for use during stable, nonemergency conditions.[14] The reality is that during complex emergencies, especially those occurring in developing countries, providers other than physicians may be providing care to children in need. Although most of the guidelines that do exist are written for physicians, many physicians are unprepared to triage a large number of pediatric patients during an emergency.[70] Moreover, there is no standardized course in pediatric disaster management.[15]

In addition to the challenges posed by the unique physical and developmental needs of children, a disproportionately small number of pediatric beds as compared with the total number of adult beds, the difficulties in accurately predicting surge capacity, and the lack of a comprehensive single source of guidelines for the care of children in complex emergencies, personal health records are not widely integrated, which if assimilated would facilitate information sharing, improve quality, and augment patient safety.[71] Yet another challenge that affects the number of available providers during complex emergencies is the lack of universal multistate credentialing for nurses, physicians, respiratory therapists, or other providers who may be available to respond during a disaster.[57] It is difficult to anticipate every situation that may occur during a complex emergency involving children,[16] thus emphasizing the critical importance of preplanning.

BEFORE A COMPLEX EMERGENCY
The Disaster is in the Details...Planning, Planning, and More Planning

Leaders and leadership are integral to successful emergency preparedness[72,73] and the effectiveness of a network.[9] Communication, collaboration, and coordination among all local and regional resources is essential to respond effectively in an emergency and meet the unique needs of children.[10,22,57,64,74–77] Because it is likely that complex emergencies will indeed include children, including pediatricians,[22,35,57,64] primary care providers, school officials,[74] prehospital responders,[64] in addition to public and private entities[18] and payers[9,74] in planning for disasters will facilitate effective relationships and promote the protection of children.[9]

Establishing a disaster resource center, which includes necessary personal protective equipment, pediatric specific supplies, and decontamination equipment, is recommended.[15] Schools should maintain equipment and resources necessary to respond to an emergency.[78] Because there may be hundreds if not thousands of children present during an emergency, both communities and schools must be prepared for an event that may last for hours if not days.[74] The emergency management planning guidelines developed for schools,[79] if used in conjunction with established disaster plans, may complement the efforts of local and regional responders.[35] In addition, maintaining a stockpile of pediatric supplies in both pediatric and primary care physicians' offices may assist in meeting the needs of those children without life-threatening conditions during a complex emergency.[20]

Anticipate Surge Capacity

Although predicting the exact number of beds needed to accommodate a surge of pediatric disaster victims is difficult if not impossible, estimating the surge capacity of local and regional hospitals prior to a disaster is highly recommended.[18,80] Surge capacity is defined as a hospital's, a system's, or a region's ability to effectively handle a sudden or rapidly increasing number of patients with a set amount of resources at a particular point in time.[81] The federal surge target is 500 adult and pediatric patients per million population in a disaster,[61] but may actually be closer to 100 to 300 adult and pediatric patients per million population for trauma or burns.[82] Others recommend preparing for a 300% increase in capacity.[83] Of the total number of pediatric patients requiring care during disasters, up to 30% may require critical care.[84] Indeed, pediatric critical care beds are most likely to be exhausted early on during an emergency, and prove the most difficult to add,[60,63] further eroding surge capacity. Determining surge capacity at local and regional schools to handle first aid and minor needs[74] may help to offset the number of children at acute care hospitals, thus improving surge capacity.

Educate, Educate, Educate

Pediatricians and primary care physicians play an important role in educating families about disaster and emergency preparedness.[20,35,85] Families who discuss disaster and emergency readiness with their primary care physicians tend to be more compliant with disaster preparedness recommendations.[86] Evidence suggests that children may cope better with disasters if they are included in preparing for disasters with their family.[27]

Providing anticipatory education to parents about the importance of preparing a personal health information worksheet for every member of the family,[87] in addition to taking along any necessary medication, and ensuring that each child has identification should evacuation or separation become necessary is recommended.[57] Children with special needs are especially vulnerable during complex emergencies, and require additional and focused planning. Personal health information, medical records, a medical alert bracelet, and identification tags are critical to the safety of these children, especially if they must evacuate, with or without their family.[57] To maintain safety and continuity of necessary medical or nursing care, some children with special needs may require transport out of the area if emergent conditions are anticipated,[64] as was seen during Hurricane Katrina.[88] For children's safety and protection, it is emphasized that parent-child separation should be avoided unless absolutely necessary to receive medical care.

Parents also need anticipatory education about children's age and developmentally specific reactions to disasters or emergency conditions.[85] Younger children may exhibit crying, fear, difficulty in communicating or sleeping, or behavior consistent with an earlier age, such as bedwetting. In addition to exhibiting some of the same behaviors of younger children, school-age and older children may also exhibit anger, aggression, withdrawal, or risk-taking behaviors. It is not unusual for children experiencing disaster conditions to become preoccupied with details of the event.[1,89]

Violence and crime may increase during disasters. Children who witness violence or death may be at increased risk of posttraumatic reactions.[33] Due to the potential long-term physical and psychological impact to the children who experience or witness disasters, training is especially important for those caregivers, whether they are parents, teachers, social workers, or health care providers, who support children both during and in the aftermath of a disaster.[90,91]

Critical preplanning elements include considering the unique physical, developmental, and psychosocial needs of children,[9,15] as well as educating prehospital and disaster response teams about age-, size-, and weight-specific assessment parameters, pediatric assessment and triage tools, and the need for pediatric-specific equipment and drug dosages.[15,18] Ideally, evidence-based pediatric guidelines that have been adapted for the geographic region and for the scope and skill of the provider are needed.[14,30,92]

We Play Like We Practice...Time for Dress Rehearsal

Simulation exercises and disaster drills are needed to practice communication and coordination among families and responders.[15,64] Simulation exercises improve readiness and promote a more coordinated response to emergencies,[18,93] and should be included in disaster planning.[16] Performing simulation exercises in teams and regions improves performance of responders and teams.[15,94,95]

DURING A COMPLEX EMERGENCY
One Size Doesn't Fit All...Triage and Treat Appropriately

During disasters or complex emergencies, the needs of pediatric victims are different from those of adult victims. Age-, size-, and weight-specific equipment and medications should be available and employed by specially trained prehospital responders.[19] Pediatric specific prehospital triage tools can aid in responding to the needs of child victims during a disaster. An example of a pediatric-specific triage tool is JumpSTART, which was derived from START, an adult prehospital triage tool.[70] Another example is the Pediatric Assessment Triangle, developed by the American Academy of Pediatrics in 2000, for use during prehospital triage and care of children during a mass-casualty event.[96] Decontamination procedures should be reviewed and altered to address the physical differences inherent in the pediatric population.[18]

Distribute Children to Control Surge

To accommodate as many pediatric patients as possible during a disaster, surge must be controlled.[60,63,97] Optimizing pediatric surge depends on excellent communication among interdisciplinary emergency responders and hospital teams about a hospital's capacity and the availability of transportation, potentially to hospitals remote from the disaster area.[57,80] Pediatric surge capacity is exceeded when the need for people, supplies, equipment, and beds necessary for the care of pediatric disaster victims exceeds the supply.[57]

Several strategies have been recommended to control surge, thus optimizing the number of available pediatric beds and reducing the premature exhaustion of pediatric supplies and providers. One strategy to control surge is to preferentially distribute pediatric patients who are more stable to sites remote from the disaster area. Doing so preserves capacity for those critically injured children.[57,60] Another strategy to control surge is to avoid using beds in hospitals dedicated to the care of children for adult victims if at all possible.[60]

During complex emergencies, expanding pediatric capacity may be necessary if the number of pediatric patients exceeds the number of pediatric supplies and beds available. Through discretionary discharges, increasing the scope of professional practice,[84] conserving supplies, exercising prudent judgment in ordering radiologic and laboratory tests, reducing the burden of documentation, and using standing orders, surge capacity may be increased.[60,63] Controlling pediatric surge and, when indicated, altering the standards of care to expand pediatric capacity during a large-scale disaster may reduce mortality rates[97,98] in a mass disaster situation.

Meeting Basic Needs Whether Children are Sheltered in Place, or Evacuated

Actions comparable to those recommended to reduce disease and death, as well as improving the overall health of children worldwide are especially relevant during disasters, because the conditions are much the same. During disasters, much like the everyday conditions in developing countries, there is often no electricity, no clean or running water, little food, inadequate shelter or clothing, and little to nothing available with which to keep clean. In addition, there may be an interruption in medical supplies, such as vaccines and antibiotics. Having access to nutritious food,[99] clean, covered water,[100] soap,[101] bed nets, vaccines, and antibiotics reduce morbidity and mortality in children during and in the aftermath of disasters.[102] Evacuation facilities should provide for personal space to the extent possible, privacy, and protection.[57,103]

Parents are the best source of support and protection for children in a disaster.[27] Children take their cues about how to react or respond to a situation from their parents. Parents may be able to reduce their child's anxiety and promote adaptive coping by controlling their own reactions to the situation. Children are at increased risk if separated from their parents during or after a disaster. The children at greatest risk are those children with disabilities or special needs who experience a sudden disaster.[32] Therefore, separating children from their parents should be avoided unless it is absolutely necessary.[18,57,103]

Having access to children's personal health information and medical records, whether portable in hard copy, or ideally, in an electronic, integrated format, facilitates information sharing among providers, thus promoting continuity of care and patient safety. This information is particularly important for those children with special needs or disabilities, or for those who have been evacuated.[71,104-106] For example, being able to connect to the Louisiana Immunization Network following Hurricane Katrina helped pediatric providers in Houston-Harris County, Texas avoid administering duplicate and unnecessary vaccinations, thus reducing expenses.[107]

IN THE AFTERMATH OF A COMPLEX EMERGENCY
Reunite Children with Their Parents as Soon as Possible

Children who are separated from their parents during a disaster, especially those separated unintentionally, are at highest risk of death.[41] Most, if not all unaccompanied children are not prepared to meet their own needs, and need protection from people who may exploit, abuse, or abduct them.[102] All agencies involved in disasters must know the plan for reuniting children with their parents if separation is unavoidable.[64,89]

Resume Routine and Restore Normalcy

Due to their unique developmental characteristics and needs, children need support and structure in the aftermath of a disaster. It is important to restore as much routine and normalcy as possible, as soon as possible following a disaster. Allowing younger children to play and resuming school for older children is constructive, promotes adaptive coping, and facilitates recovery. School also provides access to peers, an important source of support for school-age children.[74,102]

Monitoring and limiting exposure to the media,[108,109] communicating simply and honestly, and listening and clarifying misunderstanding may help children process the event.[102] Because it is common for children to fear a repetition of the event, separation from caregivers, or additional loss, it is important to encourage communication, share fears, and provide praise and frequent reassurance.[27,102] Allowing children to participate in recovery efforts and in helping to rebuild after a disaster also promotes adaptive coping.[102]

Support for Children and Parents

Evidence suggests that disasters negatively affect mental health.[110–115] Studies revealed an increase in mental health problems among people affected by Gulf Coast storms.[115] It has been found that even those children within a 160-km radius of an event but not directly affected by it may need psychological screening and support.[92] Due to inherent physical and developmental differences, children, especially those with disabilities or special needs, may experience a more difficult recovery following a disaster or complex emergency.[116] Children at highest risk for maladaptive coping and ineffective recovery in the aftermath of a disaster are those with a prior history of a psychiatric condition.[89]

A child's ability to cope during and in the aftermath of a disaster is influenced by parent or caregiver coping,[117,118] as well as the severity of the disaster, predisaster functioning, socioeconomic status, and the availability of psychosocial resources.[29] Complex emergencies and disasters affect parents' ability to provide for needs.[119] Being unable to meet children's needs in a disaster creates parental or caregiver stress. Increased parental or caregiver stress may negatively affect parenting, and may increase the potential for posttraumatic stress disorder in children.[119,120] Family cohesion also influences children's ability to cope with stressful events.[121] Evidence suggests that too much family cohesion transmits stress from family member to family member, while too little cohesion does not help children process the stress related to disaster conditions.[117]

Children often do not voluntarily share their feelings or fears.[122] Therefore it is important to observe children for evidence of maladaptive coping, ineffective recovery, or signs and symptoms of posttraumatic stress.[89,123] Parents or caregivers should ask specifically about feelings of stress or fear.[124] Parents or caregivers are encouraged to seek help from family, social support networks,[102] and qualified professional counselors as needed.[74] Too few mental health workers in any given region during stable times, much less during disasters or complex emergencies, pose significant challenges in meeting the psychosocial needs of children and their parents.[114,125]

SUMMARY AND RECOMMENDATIONS FOR FUTURE RESEARCH

Whether disasters or complex emergencies are human-made or naturally occurring, they will continue to occur at unpredictable intervals. Success in dealing with them will depend on adequate preparation, communication, collaboration, and cooperation among both public and private entities; and using evidence-based, age-appropriate, and regionally adapted guidelines that are specific to the unique physical, developmental, and psychosocial characteristics of children. Legislative support for developing a single source of evidence-based guidelines that can improve the care for children in disaster and emergency situations is recommended,[19] as well as ways to integrate critically important medical history into broadly accessible electronic medical records.[57] Future research is needed to test the efficacy of evidence-based pediatric-specific guidelines for use in complex emergencies,[14,30] to identify

Table 1
Keeping PEDIATRICS in disaster management

	Before	During	Aftermath
P	Partner with local agencies Prepare personal health records	Protect children Provide for basic needs (food, water, toileting, shelter) Praise coping with event Parents	Protect children Provide basic needs (food, water, toileting, shelter) Peers (need support) Promote adaptive coping Play
E	Empower families & children Equipment (age-specific) Educate providers, families, and kids	Electronic medical record Equipment appropriate for children	Electronic medical record
D	Determine pediatric surge capacity (hospitals and schools)	Distribute pediatric patients to control surge Do not separate from parent	Developmentally appropriate support
I	Include pediatricians, primary care providers, schools, and payers in planning	Integrated communication	Integrated communication
A	Allow children to participate in planning	Activate integrated incident command	Activate integrated record/ information Allow children to participate in rebuilding
T	Train together	Triage kids using pediatric specific tool	Talk about it with the kids Therapy proactively
R	Rehearse plan	Respond as well coordinated, multi-agency teams Remain calm Reassure	Reunite children with parents Respect parental perceptions and feelings Resume routine ASAP Reduce exposure to media Remain calm Recognize PTSD & refer as needed
I	Identification for children	Information: regarding PHR and medical history Identification for children	Involve children in rebuilding Innovation Identification for children
C	Credential providers proactively so can legally practice either during or after	Communicate Collaborate Cooperate	Clarify misinformation
S	Stock pediatric supplies Simplify reimbursement processes	Support	Screen for maladaptive coping School ASAP Share stories & feelings

Developed from a review of referenced materials.
Abbreviations: ASAP, as soon as possible; PHR, personal health records; PTSD, posttraumatic stress disorder.

evidence-based mental health interventions for individuals versus population,[114] and determine how and when to intervene to decrease maladaptive coping in families.[126] Keeping PEDIATRICS in disaster planning, response, and recovery efforts will improve the outcomes of children who experience complex emergencies. The reader is referred to **Table 1** for a summary of recommendations.

REFERENCES

1. International Strategy for Disaster Reduction. 2010. Available at: http://www. unisdr.org/disaster-statistics/introduction.htm. Accessed August 22, 2010.
2. Penrose A, Takaki M. Children's rights in emergencies and disasters. Lancet 2006;367:698–9.
3. Arnold JL. Disaster medicine in the 21st century: future hazards, vulnerabilities, and risk. Prehosp Disaster Med 2002;17(1):3–11.
4. Bartlett S. The implications of climate change for children in lower-income countries. Children, Youth and Environments 2008;18(1):71–98.
5. Waisman Y, Aharonson-Daniel L, Mor M, et al. The impact of terrorism on children: a 2-year experience. Prehosp Disaster Med 2003;18(3):242–8.
6. Cutter SL, Boruff BJ, Shirley WL. Social vulnerability to environmental hazards. Soc Sci Q 2003;84:242–61.
7. Wisner B, Blaikie P, Cannon T, et al. At risk: natural hazards, people's vulnerability, and disasters. 2nd edition. New York: Routledge; 2004.
8. World Health Organization. Disability, including prevention, management, and rehabilitation. Geneva (Switzerland): World Health Organization; 2005.
9. Ginter PM, Wingate MS, Rucks AC, et al. Creating a regional pediatric medical disaster preparedness network: imperatives and issues. Matern Child Health J 2006;10:391–6.
10. Markenson D, Redlener I. Pediatric terrorism preparedness national guidelines and recommendations: findings of an evidence-based consensus process. Biosecur Bioterror 2004;2(4):301–19.
11. Redlener I, Markenson D. Disaster and terrorism preparedness: what pediatricians need to know. Adv Pediatr 2003;50:1–37.
12. World Health Organization. Psychological consequences of disasters: prevention and management. Geneva (Switzerland): World Health Organization; 1992.
13. McFarlane AC, Norris FH. Definitions and concepts in disaster research. In: Norris FH, Galea S, Friedman MJ, et al, editors. Methods for disaster mental health research. New York: The Guilford Press; 2006. p. 3–19.
14. Moss WJ, Ramakrishnan M, Storms D, et al. Child health in complex emergencies. Bull World Health Organ 2006;84(1):58–64.
15. Cicero MX, Baum CR. Pediatric disaster preparedness. Best planning for the worst-case scenario. Pediatr Emerg Care 2008;24(7):478–81.
16. Markovitz BP. Pediatric critical care surge capacity. J Trauma 2009;67(2): S140–2.
17. Turner TJ, Barnes H, Reid J, et al. Evidence for perinatal and child health care guidelines in crisis settings: can Cochrane help? BMC Public Health 2010;10: 170.
18. Allen GM, Parrillo SJ, Will J, et al. Principles of disaster planning for the pediatric population. Prehosp Disaster Med 2007;22(6):537–40.
19. American Academy of Pediatrics. The youngest victims: disaster preparedness to meet children's needs. 2002. Available at: http://www.aap.org/disasters/pdf/ PhysiciansSheet.pdf. Accessed August 8, 2010.

20. American Academy of Pediatrics, Committee on Pediatric Emergency Medicine. Preparation for emergencies in the offices of pediatricians and pediatric primary care providers. Pediatrics 2007;120(1):200–12.

21. Dara SI, Ashton RW, Farmer JC, et al. Worldwide disaster medical response: an historical perspective. Crit Care Med 2005;33(Suppl 1):S2–6.

22. Gamble MS, Hanners RB, Lackey C, et al. Leadership and hospital preparedness: disaster management and emergency services in pediatrics. J Trauma 2009;67(2):S79–83.

23. Bernardo LM, Veenema TG. Pediatric emergency preparedness for mass gatherings and special events. Disaster Manag Response 2004;2(4): 118–22.

24. American Academy of Pediatrics, Committee on Environmental Health and Committee on Infectious Disease. Chemical-biological terrorism and its impact on children: a subject review. Pediatrics 2000;105:662–70.

25. DeVoe ER, Bannon WM, Klein TP. Post-9/11 helpseeking by New York City parents on behalf of highly exposed young children. Am J Orthopsychiatry 2006;76:167–75.

26. Fairbrother G, Stuber J, Galea S, et al. Unmet need for counseling services among children in New York City after the September 11 attacks on the world trade center: implications for pediatricians. Pediatrics 2004;113(13): 1367–74.

27. Federal Emergency Management Agency. 2010. Available at: http://www.fema.gov/rebuild/recover/copechild.shtm. Accessed August 22, 2010.

28. Hagan JF. American Academy of Pediatrics, Committee on Psychosocial Aspects of Child and Family Health; Task Force on Terrorism. Psychosocial implications of disaster or terrorism on children: a guide for the pediatrician. Pediatrics 2005;117(5 Pt 3):S458–61.

29. Norris FH, Friedman MJ, Watson PJ, et al. 60,000 disaster victims speak: part I. An empirical review of the empirical literature, 1981–2001. Psychiatry 2002; 65(3):207–39.

30. Burton A. Caring for children amidst chaos. Environ Health Perspect 2006; 114(10):A584–91.

31. Morrow BH. Identifying and mapping community vulnerability. Disasters 1999; 23(1):1–18.

32. Peek O, Stough LM. Children with disabilities in the context of disaster: a social vulnerability perspective. Child Dev 2010;81(4):1260–70.

33. O'Donnell DA, Joshi PT, Lewin SM. Training in developmental responses to trauma for child service providers. Psychiatr Serv 2007;58(1):12–4.

34. American Academy of Pediatrics, Committee on Environmental Health. Radiation disasters and children. Pediatrics 2003;111:1455–66.

35. American Academy of Pediatrics, Committee on Pediatric Emergency Medicine; American Academy of Pediatrics, Committee on Medical Liability; Task Force on Terrorism. The pediatrician and disaster preparedness. Pediatrics 2006;117(2): 560–5.

36. Brown L. Peds patients are more vulnerable in terror attack. ED Manag 2003;15: 105–6.

37. Lynch EL, Thomas TL. Pediatric chemical exposures: are we prepared? Pediatr Emerg Care 2004;20:198–208.

38. Mace SE, Sharieff G, Bern A, et al. Pediatric issues in disaster management, part 1: the emergency medical system and surge capacity. Am J Disaster Med 2010;5(2):83–93.

39. Neumayer E, Plumper T. The gendered nature of natural disasters: the impact of catastrophic events on the gender gap in life expectancy, 1981–2002. Ann Assoc Am Geogr 2007;97(3):551–66.
40. Severin PN. Pediatric disaster preparedness: what do we do next? Pediatrics 2006;118(5):2254–5.
41. Dowell SF, Toko A, Sita C, et al. Health and nutrition in centers for unaccompanied refugee children. Experience from the 1994 Rwandan refugee crisis. JAMA 1995;273:1802–6.
42. Guha-Sapir D, Panhuis WG. Conflict-related mortality: an analysis of 37 datasets. Disasters 2004;28:418–28.
43. Black RE, Morris SS, Bryce J. Where and why are 10 million children dying every year? Lancet 2003;361:2226–34.
44. Toole MJ, Waldman RJ. The public health aspects of complex emergencies and refugee situations. Annu Rev Public Health 1997;18:283–312.
45. Centers for Disease Control. Famine-affected, refugee, and displaced populations: recommendations for public health issues. MMWR Recomm Rep 1992; 41:1–76.
46. Moore PS, Marfin AA, Quenemoen LE, et al. Mortality rates in displaced and resident populations of central Somalia during 1992 famine. Lancet 1993;341: 935–8.
47. Nabeth P, Vasset B, Guerin P, et al. Health situation of refugees in eastern Zaire. Lancet 1997;349:1031–2.
48. Jamieson DJ, Meikle SF, Hillis SD, et al. An evaluation of poor pregnancy outcomes among Burundian refugees in Tanzania. JAMA 2000;283:397–402.
49. Bartlett LA, Jamieson DJ, Kahn T, et al. Maternal mortality among Afghan refugees in Pakistan, 1999-2000. Lancet 2002;359:643–9.
50. USA Today. 2001. Available at: http://usatoday.com/news/nation/2001-06-11-mcveigh-victims.htm. Accessed October 5, 2010.
51. Academic Kids. Available at: http://www.academickids.com/encyclopedia/index.php/Columbine_High_School_massacre. Accessed October 5, 2010.
52. New York Magazine. 9/11 by the numbers. 2002. Available at: http://nymag.com/news/articles/wtc/1year/numbers.htm. Accessed October 5, 2010.
53. Shapiro I, Sherman A. (2005). Essential facts about the victims of Hurricane Katrina. Center on Budget and Policy Priorities. Available at: http://www.cbpp.org/cms/?fa=view&id=658. Accessed October 5, 2010.
54. Committee on Environmental Health. Committee on Infectious Diseases. Chemical-biological terrorism and its impact on children. Pediatrics 2006;118(3): 1267–78.
55. Martin SD, Bush AC, Lynch JA. A national survey of terrorism preparedness training among pediatric, family practice, and emergency medicine programs. Pediatrics 2006;118(3):e620–6.
56. United States Census Bureau. 2009. Available at: http://factfinder.census.gov/servlet/SAFFPopulation?_submenuId=population_0&_sse=on. Accessed October 5, 2010.
57. Johnston C, Redlener I. Critical concepts for children in disasters identified by hands-on professionals: summary of issues demanding solutions before the next one. Pediatrics 2006;117(5):S458–60.
58. National Association of Children's Hospitals and Related Institutions. 2010. Available at: http://www.childrenshospitals.net/AM/Template.cfm?Section=Facts_and_Trends&TEMPLATE=/CM/ContentDisplay.cfm&CONTENTID=12693. Accessed October 5, 2010.

59. American Hospital Association. 2010. Available at: http://www.aha.org/aha/resource-center/Statistics-and-Studies/fast-facts.html. Accessed October 5, 2010.
60. Kanter RK, Moran JR. Pediatric hospital and intensive care unit capacity in regional disaster: expanding capacity by altering standards of care. Pediatrics 2007a;119(1):94–100.
61. United States Department of Health and Human Services. Health Resources and Services Administration. Fiscal year 2004 continuation guidance, National Bioterrorism Hospital Preparedness Program. Critical benchmark #2-1: surge capacity-beds. 2004.
62. Phillips S. Current status of surge research. Acad Emerg Med 2006;13:1103–8.
63. Kanter RK, Moran JR. Hospital emergency surge capacity: an empiric New York statewide study. Ann Emerg Med 2007;50(3):314–9.
64. Shirm S, Liggin R, Dick R, et al. Prehospital preparedness for pediatric mass-casualty events. Pediatrics 2007;120(4):e756–61.
65. Graham CJ, Stuemky J, Lera TA. Emergency medical services preparedness for pediatric emergencies. Pediatr Emerg Care 1993;9:329–31.
66. Seidel JS. Emergency medical services and the pediatric patient: are the needs being met? II: training and equipping emergency medical services providers for pediatric emergencies. Pediatrics 1986;78:808–12.
67. Suruda A, Vernon DD, Readin J, et al. Pre-hospital emergency medical services: a population based study of pediatric utilization. Inj Prev 1999;5(4):294–7.
68. United States Government Accountability Office. Report to Congressional Requesters. Emergency Management: most school districts have developed emergency medical plans but would benefit from additional federal guidance. Available at: http://www.gao.gov/highlights/d07609high.pdf. Accessed October 6, 2010.
69. Beltramello C, Zagaria N, Masiello L, et al. Where there is no health worker-saving children's lives in southern Sudan. Health Exchange 2002;19–22.
70. Romig L. Pediatric triage. A system to JumpSTART your triage of young patients at MCIs. JEMS 2002;27(7):52–8.
71. Healthcare Information Management and Systems Society. HIMSS personal health record definition and position statement. Chicago: Healthcare Information Management and Systems Society; 2007. Available at: http://www.himss.org/content/files/phrdefinition071707.pdf. Accessed June 10, 2010.
72. Duncan WJ, Ginter PM, Rucks AC, et al. Organizing emergency preparedness within United States public health departments. Public Health 2007;121:241–50.
73. Stoto MA. Regionalization in local public health systems: variation in rationale, implementation, and impact on public health preparedness. Public Health Rep 2008;123:441–9.
74. American Academy of Pediatrics, Council on School Health. Policy statement—disaster planning for schools. Pediatrics 2008;122(4):895–901.
75. Behney A, Briet M, Phillips C. Pediatric mass casualty: are you ready? J Emerg Nurs 2006;32:241–5.
76. Braun BI, Winerman DV, Finn NL, et al. Integrating hospitals into community emergency preparedness planning. Ann Intern Med 2006;144:799–811.
77. State of Colorado Columbine Review Commission. Report of Governor Bill Owens' Columbine Review Commission. Denver (CO): State of Colorado; 2001.
78. Bobo N, Hallenbeck P, Robinson J. Recommended minimal emergency equipment and resources for schools: National Consensus Group Report. J Sch Nurs 2003;19(3):150–6.

79. Office of Safe and Drug-Free Schools. Practical information on crisis planning: a guide for schools and communities. Washington, DC: Office of Safe and Drug-Free Schools, US Department of Education; 2004. Available at: http://www2.ed.gov/admins/lead/safety/emergencyplan/index.html. Accessed October 6, 2010.

80. Auf der Heide E. The importance of evidence-based disaster planning. Ann Emerg Med 2006;47:34–49.

81. American College of Emergency Physicians. Health care system surge capacity recognition, preparedness, and response [policy statement]. Ann Emerg Med 2005;45:239.

82. Robertson AG, Cooper DM. Disaster surge planning in Australia: measuring the immeasurable. Med J Aust 2007;186(8):388–9.

83. Rubinson L, Hick JL, Hanfling DG, et al. Definitive care for the critically ill during a disaster: a framework for optimizing critical care surge capacity: from a task force for mass critical care summit meeting, January 26–27, 2007, Chicago, IL. Chest 2008;133(Suppl 5):18S–31S.

84. Davis DP, Poste JC, Hicks T, et al. Hospital bed surge capacity in the event of a mass-casualty incident. Prehosp Disaster Med 2005;20:34–49.

85. Stuber J, Fairbrother G, Galea S, et al. Determinants of counseling for children in Manhattan after the September 11 attacks. Psychiatr Serv 2002;53(7):815–22.

86. Olympia RP, Rivera R, Heverley S, et al. Natural disasters and mass-casualty events affecting children and families: a description of emergency preparedness and the role of the primary care physician. Clin Pediatr 2010;49(7):686–98.

87. American Academy of Pediatrics. Children's health topics: disasters. 2010. Available at: http://www.aap.org/healthtopics/disasters.cfm. Accessed October 6, 2010.

88. Baldwin S, Robinson A, Barlow P, et al. Moving hospitalized children all over the southeast: interstate transfer of pediatric patients during Hurricane Katrina. Pediatrics 2006;17(5 Pt 3):S416–20.

89. Madrid PA, Grant R, Reilly MJ, et al. Challenges in meeting immediate emotional needs: short-term impact of a major disaster on children's mental health: building resiliency in the aftermath of Hurricane Katrina. Pediatrics 2006; 117(5):S448–53.

90. DeBellis MD, Baum AS, Birmaher B. Developmental traumatology: part I. biological stress symptoms. Biol Psychiatry 1999;45:1259–70.

91. McEwen BS. Effects of adverse experiences for brain structure and function. Biol Psychiatry 2000;48:721–31.

92. Smilde-van den Doel DA, Smit C, Wolleswinkel-van den Bosch JH. School performance and social-emotional behavior of primary school children before and after a disaster. Pediatrics 2006;118(5):e1311–20.

93. Ballow S, Behar S, Claudius I, et al. Hospital-based disaster preparedness for pediatric patients: how to design a realistic set of drill victims. Am J Disaster Med 2008;3(3):171–80.

94. Hsu EB, Jenckes MW, Catlett CL, et al. Effectiveness of hospital staff mass-casualty incident training methods: a critical literature review. Prehosp Disaster Med 2004;19:191–9.

95. Sweeney B, Jasper E, Gates E. Large scale urban disaster drill involving an explosion: lessons learned by an academic medical center. Disaster Manag Response 2004;2:87–90.

96. Hohenhause SM. Practical considerations for providing pediatric care in a mass casualty incident. Nurs Clin North Am 2005;40:523–33.

97. Kanter RK. Strategies to improve pediatric disaster surge response: potential mortality reduction and tradeoffs. Crit Care Med 2007;35(12):2837–42.
98. Agency for Healthcare Research and Quality. Altered standards of care in mass casualty events. AHRQ Publication No. 05-0043. Rockville (MD): Agency for Healthcare Research and Quality; 2005.
99. Collins S, Sadler K. Outpatient care for severely malnourished children in emergency relief programmes: a retrospective cohort study. Lancet 2002;360: 1824–30.
100. Roberts L, Chartier Y, Chartier O, et al. Keeping clean water clean in a Malawi refugee camp: a randomized intervention trial. Bull World Health Organ 2001; 79:280–7.
101. Peterson EA, Roberts L, Toole MJ, et al. The effect of soap distribution on diarrhoea: Nyamithuthu refugee camp. Int J Epidemiol 1998;27:520–4.
102. UNICEF. Child survival. 2009. Available at: http://volunteers.unicefusa.org/assets/pdf/campus-vcbs/child-survival-vcb-edited-8-20-09.pdf. Accessed August 22, 2010.
103. Mace SE, Sharieff G, Bern A, et al. Pediatric issues in disaster management, part 2: evacuation centers and family separation/reunification. Am J Disaster Med 2010;5(3):149–61.
104. American Academy of Pediatrics. Policy statement—using personal health records to improve the quality of health care for children. Pediatrics 2009; 124(1):403–9.
105. Institute of Medicine, Committee on Quality of Health Care in America. Crossing the quality chasm: a new health system for the 21st century. Washington, DC: National Academies Press; 2001.
106. Tang PC, Ash JS, Bates DW, et al. Personal health records: definitions, benefits and strategies for overcoming barriers to adoption. J Am Med Inform Assoc 2006;13(2):121–6.
107. Boom JA, Dragsbaek AC, Nelson CS. The success of an immunization information system in the wake of Hurricane Katrina. Pediatrics 2007;119(6): 1213–7.
108. Pfefferbaum RL, Gurwitch RH, Robertson MJ, et al. Terrorism, the media, and distress in youth. Prev Res 2003;10(2):14–6.
109. Prinstein MJ, La Greca AM, Vernberg EM, et al. Children's coping assistance: how parents, teachers, and friends help children cope after a natural disaster. J Clin Child Psychol 1996;25(4):463–75.
110. Ahern M, Kovats RS, Wilkinson P, et al. Global health impacts of floods: epidemiologic evidence. Epidemiol Rev 2005;27(1):36–46.
111. Davis L, Siegel LJ. Posttraumatic stress disorder in children and adolescents: a review and analysis. Clin Child Fam Psychol Rev 2000;3(3):135–54.
112. Freedy JR, Saladin ME, Kilpatrick DG, et al. Understanding acute psychological distress following natural disaster. J Trauma Stress 1994;7(2):257–73.
113. Norris FH, Kaniasty K, Conrad ML, et al. Placing age differences in cultural context: a comparison of the effects of age on PTSD after disasters in the United States, Mexico, and Poland. Journal of Clinical Geropsychology 2002;8(3): 153–73.
114. Schoenbaum M, Butler B, Kataoka S, et al. Promoting mental health recovery after Hurricanes Katrina and Rita: what could we have done at what cost? Arch Gen Psychiatry 2009;66(8):906–14.
115. Weisler RH, Barbee JG, Townsend MH. Mental health and recovery in the Gulf Coast after Hurricanes Katrina and Rita. JAMA 2006;296(5):585.

116. United Nations Human Settlements Programme. Enhancing urban safety and security: global report on human settlements. London: Earthscan; 2007.
117. Laor N, Wolmer L, Cohen DJ. Mother's functioning and children's symptoms 5 years after a SCUD missile attack. Am J Psychiatry 2001;158:1020–6.
118. Smith P, Perrin S, Yule W, et al. War exposure and maternal reactions in the psychological adjustment of children from Bosnia-Herzegovina. J Child Psychol Psychiatry 2001;42:395–404.
119. Kilmer RP, Gil-Rivas V. Responding to the needs of children and families after a disaster: linkages between unmet needs and caregiver functioning. Am J Orthopsychiatry 2010;80(1):135–42.
120. Gil-Rivas V, Holman EA, Silver RC. Adolescent vulnerability following the September 11th terrorist attacks: a study of parents and their children. Appl Dev Sci 2004;8:130–42.
121. Laor N, Wolmer L, Mayes LC, et al. Israeli preschoolers under scud missile attacks: a developmental perspective on risk-modifying factors. Arch Gen Psychiatry 1996;53:416–23.
122. Wolfe DA, Sas L, Wekerle C. Factors associated with the development of post traumatic stress disorder among child victims of sexual abuse. Child Abuse Negl 1994;18:37–50.
123. Kar N, Mohapatra PK, Nayak KC, et al. Post-traumatic stress disorder in children and adolescents one year after a super-cyclone in Orissa, India: exploring cross-cultural validity and vulnerability factors. BMC Psychiatry 2007;7:8.
124. Cohen JA. American Academy of Child and Adolescent Psychiatry: practice parameters for the assessment and treatment of post-traumatic stress disorder in children and adolescents. J Am Acad Child Adolesc Psychiatry 1998; 37(Suppl 10):4S–26S.
125. New Freedom Commission on Mental Health. Achieving the promise: transforming mental health care in America final report. Rockville (MD): DHHS; 2003. Pub. No. SMA-03-3832. Available at: http://www.mentalhealthcommission.gov/reports/reports.htm. Accessed October 5, 2010.
126. Pfefferbaum B, North CS. Children and families in the context of disasters: implications for preparedness and response. Fam Psychol 2008;24(2):6–10.

Responding to the Psychosocial Needs of Children and Families in Disasters

John S. Murray, PhD, RN*

KEYWORDS

• Children • Disasters • Psychosocial needs • Nursing

In 2010, global disasters from record-breaking floods and tornados in the United States to the devastating earthquakes in Haiti, Chile, and China provide clear examples of our common vulnerability in the wake of catastrophic events. Disaster scientists predict that high numbers of natural disasters will continue in the next decade.[1] Such catastrophic events serve as a powerful stimulus for health care organizations, emergency planners, and governments to examine response preparation to disasters of immense magnitude.[2] Disasters also underscore the continued need for comprehensive resources addressing the psychosocial needs of children and families. Recent literature suggests that most health care professionals feel ill prepared to address the mental health concerns of children during disaster and to recognize the importance of bringing into focus the distinct needs of children during disaster response.[3–6]

PEDIATRIC VULNERABILITIES IN DISASTERS

Unique physiologic, anatomic, developmental, and psychosocial considerations of children as well as patterns of concentration within schools and day care settings place children at greater risk during disasters.[5,7,8] Physiologic and anatomic distinctions put children at a larger threat for traumatic injury. Small body frames, less connective tissue flexibility, and immature skeletal systems place children at an increased danger for injury to internal organs caused by flying debris from hurricanes and tornados, falling rubble from earthquakes, or fast-moving wreckage from raging flood waters. Children also have a distinctive respiratory physiology, which places them at a greater danger for inhaling biologic and chemical agents as well as dust particles from collapsed structures. Faster respiratory rates in children mean greater

The author has nothing to disclose.
Children's Hospital Boston, 300 Longwood Avenue, Boston, MA 02115, USA
* 11710 Old Georgetown Road, Unit #328, North Bethesda, MD 20852.
E-mail address: JMurray325@aol.com

exposure to larger doses of aerosolized agents and particulate matter over a shorter period. The small size of children, which places them closer to the ground, poses significant risk for exposure to heavy lethal gases such as chlorine, anthrax spores, and sarin, which because of their weight settle closer to the ground when compared with oxygen. In addition, many chemical and biologic agents are absorbed through the skin. Children have more overall surface area relative to body mass, and therefore, are more likely than adults to absorb poisonous toxins.[2,3,5,8]

Pediatric disaster experts consider the psychological and psychosocial challenges for children during disaster to be more complex than the physiologic challenge.[3,8] Children often have difficulty verbalizing their feelings in relation to disaster events. Commonly, threats to their well-being and feelings of being safe interrupt the realization of normal growth and developmental milestones. Helplessness caused by the inability to feel protected may negatively affect previously established coping mechanisms, which may for the short-term become ineffective.[8] During such circumstances it is essential that those working with children and their families help them understand the event as well cope with the associated stressors.[5,9]

DEVELOPMENTAL FRAMEWORK FOR UNDERSTANDING PSYCHOSOCIAL NEEDS OF CHILDREN

A child's response to a disaster depends on several factors such as the extent of damage witnessed, loss of family members and/or pets, availability of support, and the child's age and developmental level (**Fig. 1**).[5,8,9] Understanding the effect of disaster from a developmental perspective helps responders appropriately address the unique needs of children. A social and emotional development framework helps pediatric health care professionals caring for children and families during all stages

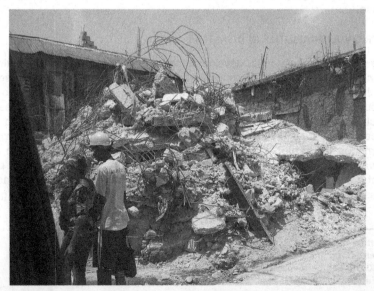

Fig. 1. Extensive damage from disasters has the potential to affect the psychosocial adaptation of children. (*Courtesy of* M. Felber, RN, Boston Children's Hospital Disaster Response Team, Boston, MA.)

of a disaster as well as to ascertain which interventions will help children to cope most effectively.[9–11]

A framework that has been found to be helpful in understanding the psychosocial needs of children under stressful conditions, such as disasters, is Erickson's framework of social and emotional development. In the first 18 months of life, infants progress through the developmental stage of trust versus mistrust. Critical during this stage is having a consistent caretaker who can be depended on to meet the infant's needs. When these needs are not met because of unavailability of the caregiver, feelings of mistrust develop.[9–13]

Young children up to the age of 3 years advance through the stage of autonomy versus shame and doubt. During this phase of development, children should be given many opportunities to be independent and self-sufficient. This milestone can be reached when caretakers encourage children to explore their environment while simultaneously ensuring that safety and security needs are met. If not given these types of opportunities, feelings such as shame and self-doubt can develop. From the ages of 3 to 6 years (preschool years), children move forward to the stage of initiative versus guilt. During this time, children endeavor to be independent of caretakers while struggling with feelings of guilt, which might arise from unplanned consequences of their actions.[9–13]

Psychosocial development from the ages of 6 to 12 years, or during middle childhood, brings in the period referred to as industry versus inferiority, which is manifested by behaviors in children aimed at mastery of life skills and challenges, which might be set by family, peers, or communities. Failure to meet this milestone can lead to feelings such as disappointment. Finally, the adolescent population progresses to the stage of identity versus role confusion. It is during this time that they search for a sense of self or identity, which sets them apart from others. During this stage, adolescents learn about their strengths and weaknesses by trying out new roles and responsibilities as well as making decisions on issues of importance. Teens who struggle with identity formation oftentimes experience troubles such as school avoidance, substance misuse, criminal activity, and other imprudent life choices. From a positive perspective, adolescents who are successful in establishing an identity during this stage show promise for positive personal growth into early adulthood.[9–13]

PSYCHOSOCIAL NEEDS IN PREPARATION FOR DISASTERS

Most of the published literature on the effects of disasters on children focuses on the aftermath. There is a dearth of literature that addresses planning for children and families in advance of a disaster from a psychosocial perspective.[3,9] Being prepared is important to helping children positively cope with disaster. Fear and panic are among the most common behaviors exhibited by children when families have not prepared for a disaster. Health care professionals and parents play an important role in preparing children for disasters by sharing age-appropriate information about disasters and guiding them on what to expect before, during, and after the event. Providing anticipatory guidance and addressing questions in advance of a disaster aids in reducing misconceptions as well as fear and anxiety.[9,14]

Pediatric disaster experts recommend that caretakers begin by determining their child's current level of knowledge regarding disasters. This information helps to determine misconceptions that the child may have regarding disasters so that information provided to the child can be better focused on meeting their informational needs. To be optimally prepared in advance of a disaster, educational materials on distinctive responses of children and adolescents to disaster should also be provided to parents and caregivers. Professional organizations such as the American Academy of Pediatrics (http://www.aap.org/), American Red Cross (http://www.redcross.org/), and National Child Traumatic Stress Network (http://www.nctsnet.org) have helpful resources available for families. Health care professionals should make a concerted effort to ensure widest dissemination of information in preparation for disasters.[9,10,15]

Essential to preparing children and families for disaster is developing a family response plan. Early planning helps to lessen fears, stress, and anxiety. Involving children and adolescents in the planning process makes constructive psychosocial adjustment possible. For example, children should be encouraged to assist parents with gathering supplies such as water, nonperishable food items, pet food and travel containers, flashlights, batteries, and other items such as lists of important telephone numbers, blankets or sleeping bags, and changes in clothing. Whereas planning is helpful, special attention should be taken to not cause increased worry with the preparation efforts. Even with the best planning, disasters are stressful for children and families.[9,10,15]

PSYCHOSOCIAL NEEDS DURING DISASTERS

Pediatric health care professionals have long recognized the importance of meeting the unique psychosocial needs of children across all age groups during disasters, which requires a collaborative partnership with the community so that the needs of children are met by professionals working in health care settings, schools, and day care facilities. Each of these professional groups plays a central role in ensuring that the special needs of children and families are met. Therefore, these professional groups should have an understanding of the psychosocial reactions of children to mitigate conditions that could result in panic.[5,9,10,16]

During disasters, adult caregivers of children are affected by stress just as much as the children. To meet the needs of children, adults must take care of their own needs. Every effort should be made to ensure that parents have appropriate emotional support needed to care for themselves as well as their children. Social networks using e-mail, Facebook, Twitter, or MySpace can serve to provide emotional support, when these are not disrupted during disaster. When power is disrupted, adults should seek emotional support from extended family members, neighbors, friends, church members, or professional colleagues.[9,10]

The response of infants to disasters depends on the stability of consistent caregivers to meet their needs for trust, security, and safety. Changes in predictable schedules or loss of a primary caretaker can lead to regressive behaviors and detachment. Adjustment to disaster depends on the effect of the event on caregivers and availability of these adults to meet the psychosocial needs of the infants. Signs of distress in infants include changes in sleeping and eating patterns, increased crying and irritability, separation anxiety, exaggerated startle response, and apathy.[9,16] Interventions for meeting the psychosocial needs of infants should include educating caregivers about the infant's possible behavioral reaction to disaster as well as the importance of ensuring that infants are provided with consistent predictable care. If the primary caregiver is injured because of the disaster, another parent or extended family member should provide this care. Consistency in caregiving and maintaining routines as close to normal as possible provides the essential foundation needed for psychosocial adaptation to a stressful event.[1,9–11,15–20]

Much the same as infants, toddlers depend on the availability of parents to feel protected and cared for. Whereas children in this age group may not have cognitive awareness of a disaster, they experience stress in their environment, especially if there is change in routine, their independence is limited, or they lose family members. Common behavioral responses of toddlers to disaster include changes in appetite, disrupted sleep, nightmares, and skill regression manifested as clinging behaviors, withdrawal, temper tantrums, and helplessness.[3,9,10,13,16,19]

Parents should be provided with educational materials and anticipatory guidance, which prepares them for possible behavioral changes that they may observe in their toddler. Like infants, toddlers need schedules that are predictable and dependable and need to feel assured that their basic needs will be met. This age group in particular requires stability in activities such as mealtimes, play, and sleep. Alterations in sleeping patterns on a provisional basis should be permitted, if needed, to help the toddler feel safe and secure. Interventions that promote relaxation at bedtime, such as the use of night-lights and comfort items (eg, stuffed animals and favorite blankets) music, and storytelling should be used. Children in this age group should also be encouraged to engage in play activities, which provides them with an opportunity to express emotions and feelings to better cope with the stressors of disaster.[9,10]

During the preschool years, children possess the cognitive ability to focus attention more so than younger age groups. Health care professionals and parents must pay critical attention to ascertain that children in this age group do not become preoccupied with the stressors associated with disaster.[9,10]

Preschoolers lack an understanding of cause and effect, which places them at risk for misinterpreting stressful situations as something that they may have caused, resulting in feelings of guilt.[12,13,17] Health care professionals caring for children in disasters should observe for reactions such as regression (eg, bedwetting, thumb sucking, and fear of the dark), alterations in eating and sleep patterns, anxiety, and somatic symptoms such as headaches and stomachaches.[1,9,10,20]

Preschoolers do not understand what is occurring in their environment during disaster and do not comprehend the consequences, therefore it is important for health care professionals and adult caretakers to continually provide reassurance. Explaining to children that they are not responsible for the disaster will help alleviate feelings of guilt. Parent education is a key aspect of psychosocial intervention. Parents and other adult caretakers such as babysitters, and daycare providers should be taught to recognize common behavioral reactions of preschoolers and be acquainted with interventions to assist children with positive psychosocial coping. Parents should understand that it is acceptable to allow children to regress to previously outgrown behaviors during this stressful period because regression will facilitate psychosocial adaptation. Interventions such as play and storytelling will promote expression of feelings and help to minimize stress (**Fig. 2**).[9,10]

School-aged children are increasingly able to think more concretely as they grow. However, just as other groups of children, they continue to be at risk for adjustment difficulties because of increased stress related to disaster. Behavioral reactions may manifest as preoccupation with disaster as well as fear for their own well-being and for that of their family members and friends. Other indications of stress might include refusal to attend school, withdrawal from social groups such as playmates, decreased interest in everyday activities, and worry over the events surrounding the disaster. Changes in temperament (eg, whining, aggressiveness, rebellion, and acting out) may also be noted.[9,10,13,16,19,20]

Extensive exposure to television, radio, Internet, or social media coverage of the disaster exacerbates stress reactions. Media coverage should be restricted as much as possible. However, parents and health care professionals should explain the happenings to children in an age-appropriate manner. Other interventions to help school-aged children include educating caretakers on the possible behavioral

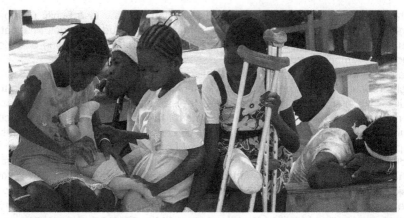

Fig. 2. Haitian children using play to express their feelings related to disaster. (*Courtesy of* M. Felber, RN, Boston Children's Hospital Disaster Response Team, Boston, MA.)

changes they might see in children. Families should provide realistic expectations of children using a structure that does not place additional stressors on children. For example, chores and household responsibilities should not be overly demanding because children strive to adapt to the stress in a positive manner. Like younger age groups, school-aged children greatly need and appreciate the opportunity to express their feelings and emotions as it relates to disaster. Several forums are available, including individual counseling with school counselors, a child psychologist supporting disaster response efforts, or groups of children who may assemble as part of group therapy. Children are better able to manage stressors related to disaster when they do not feel alone. For school-aged children who are not ready to share their feelings, expressive therapy in the form of drawing, painting, music, acting, puppet shows, or play can be beneficial in encouraging them to talk about how they are feeling.[9,14,15]

Although adolescents are the most cognitively advanced pediatric age group, they too can become overwhelmed with stress during disaster. This stress is partly related to the multifaceted changes that they are already experiencing because of their developmental stage.[9,10,13,16] Stress that goes unmanaged can lead to increased anxiety, extreme acting out, angry outburst, changes in mood, depression, emotional numbness, withdrawal, and somatic illnesses, such as headaches, stomachaches, and insomnia. Adolescents might also use poor coping strategies to manage stress, such as risk-taking behaviors including drug and alcohol abuses.[1,9,10,13,16]

Behavioral reaction of teens to disaster experiences is not all negative. Positive behaviors are also observed. Teenagers can frequently be seen helping with disaster response efforts, assuming additional responsibilities at home and providing support to family members, friends, and members of the community.[9,10,19] When safe to do so, providing this age group with additional responsibilities during disaster helps them to try out different roles, which is a key component of their developmental process. These additional roles and tasks also help them to develop positive coping skills during stress. Adolescents need an opportunity to express their feelings related to disaster like other age groups. However, they may have difficulty openly communicating their feelings.

Health care professionals and parents should provide opportunities for teens to engage in conversation with their peers whenever possible. Other options include facilitating adolescent discussions with adult mentors, coaches, school counselors, or clergy.[9,10] Additional interventions may include assisting teens to understand the effect of disaster on their behaviors and responses to the stressful situation. This intervention serves as a time to help teens become cognizant of how they handle stress as well as to explore and test various coping strategies. Coping skills that can be used include relaxation techniques, various forms of exercise to decrease stress, blogging if Internet access is available, journal writing, and participation in support groups.[9]

PSYCHOSOCIAL NEEDS AFTER DISASTERS

For children across all age groups, behavioral reactions to disaster are normal and temporary. However, some children experience ongoing adjustment difficulties that can potentially result in enduring adjustment difficulties such as posttraumatic stress disorder (PTSD). Children with PTSD present with behavioral difficulties such as emotional unresponsiveness, depression, withdrawal from social groups, and feeling separated from their own emotions. Other behavioral symptoms may include changes in sleep patterns, difficulty concentrating, irritability, anger, regression, and compulsive concentration on death. Early intervention is critical for successful resolution of psychosocial difficulties.[1,9,10,21–23] Pediatric mental health professionals play a critical role in the diagnosis and treatment of children and adolescents with PTSD. However, support from parents, extended family members, peers, schoolteachers, and community members are also paramount.[9] Additional interventions that have been found to be helpful include various forms of psychotherapy such as individual, family, or group therapy, which give a child an opportunity to talk, write, draw, or play about stressful events surrounding the disaster. Cognitive behavioral therapy, behavior modification techniques, and cognitive therapy have also been successfully used to reduce fears, establish feelings of safety, and manage symptoms in children exposed to public health emergencies such as disasters.[1,9]

The media frequently covers the all-too-common ultimate tragedy of disaster, the loss of life. With this loss, it can be expected that children and adolescents will experience significant grief. Health care professionals can play an important role in educating parents and other adult caretakers about the possible behavioral changes and adjustment difficulties that might be seen because of loss and during the grieving process, including anger, sadness, withdrawal from support systems and social groups, retreat from social activities and hobbies, decreased psychological interest in everyday activities, as well as changes in eating and sleeping patterns.[9,23] Those caring for children during disaster can also be instrumental in identifying community support resources and help with facilitating coordination of care with organizations such as churches, relief shelters, or local mental health clinic support groups. Early involvement with age-appropriate interventions is essential to identifying adjustment difficulties in children as well as to helping families assist their children to positively adjust to a difficult life situation.[9,10,22]

COLLABORATING TO HELP MEET THE PSYCHOSOCIAL NEEDS OF CHILDREN

One of the most important interventions that pediatric health care professionals can be involved in during a disaster is collaboration with the community, especially school systems and hospitals. Children across all age groups spend most of their time in school, thereby creating an important environment for health care professionals providing support and intervention during all phases of a disaster. School systems provide an optimal setting to assess the needs of children.[5,9–11] Partnering with teachers is beneficial for pediatric health care specialists, who can use the school environment as a platform for providing age-specific educational materials and recommendations on interventions for children experiencing difficulty related to disaster.

Sharing information about what to expect from children during disaster, providing suggestions on age-appropriate and culturally sensitive interventions, assisting in developing a list of referral services, and offering to provide assessments for adjustment difficulties and high-risk behaviors can result from this alliance. School districts also function as a point of intervention where pediatric behavioral health experts can provide assessments for children experiencing difficulties and offer support programs to help children adjust in a positive manner. School systems also provide health care professionals with ease of access to parents. This linkage provides an opportunity to educate parents and assist them with developing family care plans during disaster.[5,9–11,15,24]

Collaboration with hospital systems is also an important endeavor for pediatric health care professionals responding to disasters. Hospitals need to be fully prepared to care for large numbers of injured children. Health care systems must be appropriately resourced to meet the special needs of children and families. Pediatric disaster response experts have articulated the importance of having provisions for surge capacity to care for the pediatric population. This undertaking requires close partnering with local, state, and federal disaster response agencies.[9,25,26] Pediatric public health emergency plans have been published to assist health care professionals with pediatric hospital surge capacity in the event of a disaster. These guidelines serve as an exceptional resource for health care delivery systems to improve response and interventions for children and families affected by disaster.[5,25]

The media can be a powerful partner in educating communities about disaster preparation. Pediatric health care professionals should take advantage of this resource whenever possible. Media vehicles can include print in the form of newspaper or journal articles, pamphlets, and news bulletins or electronic means such as radio, television, and the Internet. Critical information can also be disseminated at community events such as town hall meetings; parent-teacher and school council meetings; gatherings at places of worship; educational offerings at neighborhood clinics; pediatric health care provider offices; as well as local, state, and federal disaster response agencies.[9–11]

IMPLICATIONS FOR CLINICAL PRACTICE, EDUCATION, TRAINING, RESEARCH, AND POLICY

Pediatric health care professionals have long played a critical role in disaster response. This responsibility grows with the increase in worldwide disasters. More than any other group, children and adolescents are at risk for adjustment difficulties. Therefore, additional work in education, training, and research is needed to improve the care delivered and subsequently to enhance clinical outcomes. A better understanding of the psychosocial needs of children and families at all stages of disaster is critically needed. Greater cognizance of the behavioral health needs will assist pediatric health care professionals with identifying the requisite resources and interventions necessary for meeting these needs during disaster. Recognizing the psychosocial needs of children and families before, during, and after disaster will assist providers of care to more accurately assess potential psychosocial stressors, including their effect. Ultimately, this assessment will enable health care professionals to provide age-appropriate, developmentally responsive, and culturally sensitive behavioral health interventions.[9,27]

Although pediatric disaster research has made some progress since the terrorist attacks of September 11, 2001, an extraordinary opportunity exists for pediatric health care providers to advance the state of the science, especially as it relates to addressing the psychosocial needs of children and families. Research on the psychosocial implications of disaster on children remains largely unexplored; therefore, an expanded research agenda in the area of pediatric disaster preparedness and response is critically needed. Some progress has been made to guide child-focused disaster research using conceptual models; however, more effort is needed to further develop and evaluate this aspect of research. In addition, an understanding of the effects of disaster on children and families is needed. Just as essential is the need to critically evaluate and test interventions for pediatric survivors of disaster and their families. Whereas most research has focused on the postdisaster period, greater efforts need to be directed toward intervention research before and during disasters. Disaster researchers are increasingly mindful of the significant need to continue to advance the state of the science of the effects of disasters on children and families, which will bring about positive psychosocial adjustment for those experiencing the numerous stressors associated with catastrophic events.[9,11,27]

Finally, unlike any other time in history, an incredible opportunity exists for pediatric health care professionals to affect policy related to disaster response focused on meeting the psychosocial needs of children and families. Other investigators have highlighted the critical need for health care providers to advocate and lead initiatives to improve the care of children and families throughout all stages of disaster. Greater attention must be focused on raising public awareness regarding the needs of children during disaster. Better sources of funding for research are needed to improve the state of the science regarding the full effect that disasters have on children. A concerted effort is needed to teach health care professionals from all disciplines about the distinct behavioral health needs of children and adolescents. Such education can be provided as part of graduate education or through continuing education programs offered by professional organizations. Finally, every institution that provides care or services for children should have age-appropriate disaster response plans and intervention protocols available including content addressing the psychological needs of children and adolescents in disaster. Health policy is fundamental to enhancing the ability of health care professionals to appropriately respond to disaster across the continuum.[9,24,25,27]

SUMMARY

Pediatric health care professionals play a critical role in disaster response by assisting parents, teachers, and health care organizations to meet the unique needs of children, adolescents, and families during all phases of disaster. Addressing the psychosocial needs of this vulnerable population by providing age-appropriate care and facilitating adaptive coping strategies has the potential to decrease the long-term behavioral health consequences and help children positively adjust to a stressful life experience.

REFERENCES

1. Baggerly J, Exum H. Counseling children after natural disasters: guidance for family therapists. Am J Fam Ther 2008;36:79–93.
2. Markenson H, Krug S. Developing pediatric emergency preparedness performance measures. Clin Ped Emer Med 2009;10:229–39.

3. Shonfeld D, Gurwitch R. Addressing disaster mental health needs of children: practical guidance for pediatric emergency health care providers. Clin Ped Emer Med 2009;10:208–14.
4. Shannon M, Baum K. Pediatric preparedness for disasters: where are we now? Current challenges and future directions. Clin Ped Emer Med 2009; 10:128–9.
5. Murray J. Public health emergencies and children: new guidelines offer an opportunity to be better prepared. Am J Nurs 2009;109:28–31.
6. Institute of Medicine (IOM). Future of emergency care: emergency care for children, growing pains. Washington, DC: The National Academies Press; 2006.
7. Mason K, Anderson M. Challenges facing pediatric preparedness. Clin Ped Emer Med 2009;10:159–61.
8. Fendya D. When disaster strikes: care considerations for pediatric patients. J Trauma Nurs 2006;13:161–5.
9. Murray J. A collaborative approach to meeting the psychosocial needs of children during an influenza pandemic. J Spec Pediatr Nurs 2010;15:135–43.
10. Murray J. Addressing the psychosocial needs of children following disasters. J Spec Pediatr Nurs 2006;11:133–7.
11. Murray J. Understanding the effects of disaster on children: a developmental-ecological approach to scientific inquiry. J Spec Pediatr Nurs 2006;15: 199–202.
12. Child Development Institute. Stages of social-emotional development in children and teenagers. Available at: http://www.childdevelopmentinfo.com/development/erickson.shtml. Accessed May 12, 2010.
13. Feldman R. Development across the life span. 5th edition. New Jersey: Prentice Hall; 2007. p. 18, 203, 259, 347, 420–421.
14. American Academy of Pediatrics. Family readiness kit: preparing to handle disaster. Available at: http://www.aap.org/family/frk/frkit.htm. Accessed May 12, 2010.
15. American Psychological Association. Strengthening your emotional well being ahead of the flood. Available at: http://www.apa.org/helpcenter/flood-preparation.aspx. Accessed May 12, 2010.
16. Hagan Jr JF, The Committee on Psychosocial Aspects of Child and Family Health, The Task Force on Terrorism. Psychosocial implications of disaster or terrorism on children: a guide for the pediatrician. Pediatrics 2005;116:787–95.
17. Murray J. Helping children cope with separation during war. J Spec Pediatr Nurs 2002;7:127–30.
18. Zubenko W. Developmental issues in stress and crisis. In: Zubenko WN, Capozzoli JA, editors. Children and disasters: a practical guide to healing and recovery. New York: Oxford University Press; 2002. p. 85–100.
19. Plum K. Understanding the psychosocial impact of disasters. In: Veenema TG, editor. Disaster nursing and emergency preparedness for chemical, biological, and radiological terrorism. New York: Springer; 2003. p. 68–9.
20. Becker S. Psychosocial care for adult and child survivors of the tsunami disaster in India. J Child Adolesc Pscyh Nurs 2007;20:148–55.
21. La Greca A, Prinstein M. Hurricanes and earthquakes. In: La Greca A, Silverman W, Vernberg E, et al, editors. Helping children cope with disasters and terrorism. Washington, DC: American Psychological Association; 2002. p. 119–21.
22. Emergency Medical Services for Children. After the emergency is over: post-traumatic stress disorder in children and youth. Available at: http://bolivia.hrsa.gov/emsc/downloads/ptsd/PTSD.pdf. Accessed May 12, 2010.

23. American Academy of Child and Adolescent Psychiatry. Helping children after a disaster. Available at: http://www.aacap.org/publications/factsfam/disaster.htm. Accessed May 12, 2010.
24. Chung S, Danielson J, Shannon M. School-based emergency preparedness: a national analysis and recommended protocol. Available at: http://www.ahrq.gov/prep/schoolprep/. Accessed May 12, 2010.
25. Boyer E, Fitch J, Shannon M. Pediatric hospital surge capacity in public health emergencies. Available at: http://www.ahrq.gov/prep/pedhospital/. Accessed May 12, 2010.
26. Shonfeld D. Mental health concerns. Clin Ped Emer Med 2009;10:153–5.
27. La Greca A, Silverman W, Vernberg E, et al. Children and disasters: future directions for research and public policy. In: La Greca A, Silverman W, Vernberg E, et al, editors. Helping children cope with disasters and terrorism. Washington, DC: American Psychological Association; 2002. p. 405–20.

Disaster Planning for Vulnerable Populations: Mental Health

Thomas B. Mendez, PhD(c), MSN, RN, CNS*

KEYWORDS

• Mental health • Disasters • Preparedness • Nursing

There is evidence to suggest that society has dealt with the ramifications of disasters since the beginning of recorded time. Worldwide communication systems have resulted in moment-by-moment opportunities to witness the horrifying outcomes of catastrophic events on populations. Recent events such as the terrorist acts on September 11, 2000, tsunami in 2004 that struck Southeast Asia, Hurricane Katrina on August 28, 2005 (in which an estimated 1800 people were killed, causing $81 billion of damage), and Hurricane Ike on September 13, 2008 (reportedly causing 195 deaths and $22 billion of damage) have brought critically needed attention to the significance of disaster planning and emergency preparedness.

One of the most devastating disasters in recent times is the earthquake in Haiti January 2010, which killed an estimated 330,000 people and displaced 1.5 million inhabitants. A 2010 study by the Inter-American Development Bank notes that in addition to the astounding loss of life and life-altering nature of the injuries sustained by the survivors, the total cost of the disaster was between $8 billion and $14 billion, making it one of the most destructive natural disasters of modern time.[1] Most of Haiti's infrastructure, including medical facilities, were either damaged or destroyed during the quake, leaving the masses without much in the way of basic necessities, including food, water, hygiene, and medical care. Given the amount of destruction, concerns about the day-to-day existence for the most resilient survivors underscore the implications for vulnerable populations in the aftermath of disasters of this magnitude.

Based on the experiences of past disasters, there is a plethora of information that addresses the psychological effect on survivors after a disaster. The Centers for Disease Control and Prevention (CDC) has developed guiding principles (**Fig. 1**) that

The author has nothing to disclose.
School of Nursing, 3.526 Allied Health Sciences/Nursing Building, 301 University Boulevard, Galveston, TX 77555-0129, USA
* School of Health Professions, University of Texas Medical Branch, 301 University Boulevard, Mail Route 1029, Galveston, TX 77555-0144.
E-mail address: tbmendez@utmb.edu

Crit Care Nurs Clin N Am 22 (2010) 493–500
doi:10.1016/j.ccell.2010.10.001   ccnursing.theclinics.com

Guiding Principles: Mental Health Related Emergency Preparedness and Response

- No one who experiences a disaster is untouched by it.

- Most people pull together and function during and after a disaster, but their effectiveness is diminished.

- Mental health concerns exist in most aspects of preparedness, response and recovery.

- Disaster stress and grief reactions are "normal responses to an abnormal situation."

- Survivors respond to active, genuine interest and concern.

- Disaster mental health assistance is often more practical than psychological in nature (offering a phone, distributing coffee, listening, encouraging, reassuring, comforting).

- Disaster relief assistance may be confusing to disaster survivors. They may experience frustration, anger, and feelings of helplessness related to Federal, State, and non-profit agencies' disaster assistance programs. They may reject disaster assistance of all types.

Fig. 1. Guiding principles: mental health–related emergency preparedness and response. (*From* Centers for Disease Control and Prevention. Disaster mental health primer: key principles, issues and questions. Available at: http://www.bt.cdc.gov/mentalhealth/primer.asp. Accessed July 10, 2010.)

provide the concepts to be considered when preparing for or responding to a disaster.[2] One such concept is that no individual experiencing a disaster is untouched by it. Generally, the experience includes loss, which can be real, perceived, or anticipated. Loss can include one or more elements such as the death of a loved one, loss of home, loss of employment or income, loss of independence, or loss of safety after a traumatic event. From loss comes grief, which is a multifaceted natural response to loss. Grief is individual and influenced by several factors including one's cultural and spiritual beliefs. Further complicating the process is a sudden or an unexpected loss, such as that which occurs during and after a disaster. Such a loss can surpass survivors' coping mechanisms and can lead to feelings of being powerless and overwhelmed; leaving individuals unable to function. Although people may have an understanding of what has occurred, they may not be able to comprehend the full extent of the loss and may take a longer time to understand what has occurred. Exaggerated or prolonged grief can lead to a depression and an inability to function.

Another concept noted in the guiding principles is that mental health concerns exist in most aspects of preparedness, response, and recovery.[2] Disasters are significant stressful events, and how individuals manage their stress can be greatly affected. Normal coping mechanisms may not be enough to provide support to a person under severe stress, and the effects may manifest in several physical, psychological, and emotional ways ranging from general restlessness to agitated behavior, from an increased heart rate to chest pains, from mental slowness to confusion and difficulty in concentrating, from feelings of irritation to frustration, and feelings of being overwhelmed and helpless. The relationship between stress and other health issues such as immune suppression, cardiac problems, and hypertension has been established. In addition, there is a relationship between stress and depression as well as other psychiatric disorders such as severe anxiety, posttraumatic stress disorder (PTSD), mood disorders, and schizophrenia.

The primer also identifies the phases of a disaster (**Fig. 2**), which is based on a longitudinal approach to the psychological experiences and overall effects encountered by most individuals after disaster.[2]

However, response to this process is individualized, and the period between disillusionment and reconstruction is of key importance because it includes the grief process. In the book *On Death and Dying*, Kübler-Ross[3] describes 5 stages of grief recognized as the processes followed by those grieving a loss, including the loss of a loved one. These widely accepted stages of grief include stage 1, denial; stage 2, anger; stage 3, bargaining; stage 4, depression; and stage 5, acceptance.[3] Kessler,[4] coauthor with Kübler-Ross (*On Death and Dying*) and author of *The Needs of Dying*, states, "[w]e do not enter and leave each individual stage in a linear fashion". Prolonged or exaggerated grief can lead to severe depression and an inability to function and may require professional attention.

One of the most striking figures in the CDC primer is the chart representing the severity of psychological reaction after a traumatic event (**Fig. 3**).[2] The chart demonstrates that most people affected by a disaster experience mild reactions to the event, such as insomnia, worry, and feeling upset, whereas a lesser number experience a slightly more pronounced or moderate reaction in the form of persistent insomnia and/or anxiety. Fewer in number, but to a greater extent, individuals experience severe reactions such as PTSD and depression. Severe reactions may manifest as symptoms ranging from generalized disorientation including memory loss, inability to recall recent events, and inability to recall date or time. Symptoms of depression range from a pervasive feeling of hopelessness or helplessness to total despair. Symptoms of anxiety consist of moderate to severe anxiety and may include feelings of restlessness, escalating to hypervigilance and/or obsessive fear of another disaster. Other psychiatric and mental health symptoms include suicidal or homicidal thoughts or plans, inability to care for self, including eating, bathing, or other activities of daily living. Psychotic symptoms include auditory and visual hallucinations and delusional thinking. Excessive use of alcohol or drugs, domestic violence, and child or elder abuse may be the symptoms.

VULNERABLE POPULATION

An area not well addressed in the literature is that of emergency preparedness and disaster planning for a person with a psychiatric and mental health need before

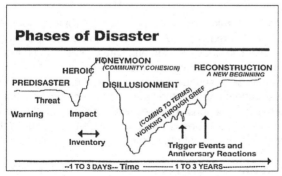

Fig. 2. Phases of disaster. (*From* Centers for Disease Control and Prevention. Disaster mental health primer: key principles, issues and questions. Available at: http://www.bt.cdc.gov/mentalhealth/primer.asp. Accessed July 10, 2010.)

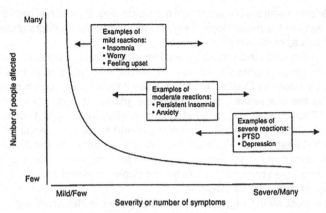

Fig. 3. Severity of psychological reaction after a traumatic event. (*From* Centers for Disease Control and Prevention. Disaster mental health primer: key principles, issues and questions. Available at http://www.bt.cdc.gov/mentalhealth/primer.asp. Accessed July 10, 2010.)

a catastrophic event. Much is published on the importance of addressing the mental health needs of those affected by a disaster; however, little has been published regarding those with existing psychiatric and mental health issues.

According to the National Alliance on Mental Illness[5] (2010), "[e]ven though mental illness is widespread in the population, the main burden of illness is concentrated in a much smaller proportion – about 6 percent, or 1 in 17 Americans who live with a serious mental illness". The National Institute of Mental Health[6] (2010) reports that an estimated 26.2% of Americans 18 years and older, or 1 in 4 adults, have a diagnosable mental disorder in a given year. The United States Department of Health and Human Services, Substance Abuse and Mental Health Services Administration's (SAMHSA) National Mental Health Information Center (2010) notes that psychiatric and mental health factors such as untreated mental illness, substance abuse, and co-occurring disorders are individual factors that can increase an individual's risk for becoming homeless and remaining homeless for longer periods. Of an estimated 842,000 adults and children who are homeless in a given week, 38% report alcohol use problems; 26% report other drug use problems; 39% report some form of psychiatric or mental health problem and 20% to 25% meet the criteria for serious mental illness; and 66% report substance use and/or mental health problems.[7]

The National Mental Health Information Center[7] (2010) also notes that symptoms are often active and untreated, making it difficult for those with mental health problems to meet the basic needs for food, shelter, and safety, thus being a significant factor in the relationship between mental illness and homelessness. In addition, the report notes that individuals with serious mental illnesses have greater difficulty exiting homelessness than others and that they are more often homeless for longer periods than other homeless populations. Coupled with obstacles such as homelessness, individuals with mental health needs become an even more vulnerable population; this is particularly true in the event of a disaster.[7]

PARALLEL POPULATION

While not specific to mental health, issues affecting the vulnerable elderly during disasters are applicable to the population with mental health needs as well. In 2008,

Dosa and colleagues[8] identified and discussed major concerns inherent in the management of another vulnerable population affected by a disaster, the elderly nursing home resident population. The primary focus of the article centers on the numerous deaths of nursing home residents that occurred during Hurricanes Katrina and Rita. The investigators identified several factors that complicate the safe evacuation of the nursing home resident, such as frailty, lack of mobility, dementia, or vision/hearing difficulties that complicate the evacuation process. Another important factor identified is the increased acuity of nursing home residents, due in part to shorter lengths of stay in acute care facilities, compounded by complex cardiac and orthopedic issues that increase the overall vulnerability of the population. The investigators also noted the potential high risk for exacerbation of psychiatric diseases, such as PTSD, depression, and anxiety. In addition, the presence of cognitive impairments and disruption of daily life caused by disaster-related activities have the potential to further affect psychiatric-related issues.

A fundamental question noted in the research centers on whether to evacuate or not.[8] Analyses of data from Hurricanes Katrina, Rita, and Wilma have shown that the question is extremely complex and not easily answered. Issues such as evacuating and transporting frail adults and the inability of temporary shelters to accommodate the functional and physical needs of the elderly were identified. A separate pilot study of 20 Louisiana nursing homes for the Kaiser Family Foundation identified large-scale problems associated with evacuation that further validated the overwhelming task of evacuation of nursing home residents.[9] In the pilot study, 9 nursing home administrators who decided to evacuate residents reported experiencing greater problems than those who decided to shelter the residents in place. After phone interviews with the administrators and follow-up group sessions, 2 central themes were identified: (1) administrators felt abandoned by local, state, and federal emergency preparedness officials and (2) there was a substantial physical and technical difficulty evacuating nursing home residents. Similarly, coordination of emergency needs with state and local governments were identified as being problematic. The investigators note that "it is plausible and indeed likely that more graduated approaches to evacuation are more effective," and more research is indicated. In addition, it is suggested that one approach to determine whether to evacuate all residents, select residents, or to shelter in place can be viewed "as a summation of separate elements of person risk, facility risk, and disaster event risk". In conclusion, the investigators note that a vast majority of hurricane-associated mortality was among the elderly in Gulf State nursing homes and that many perished either because they failed to evacuate or because of complications caused by poorly executed evacuations. The unique needs of nursing home residents must be incorporated into existing and future governmental emergency response systems. Many of the issues identified and lessons learned in these studies can be applied to populations with mental health needs.

CRITICAL INCIDENT STRESS DEBRIEFING

Critical incident stress debriefing or crisis intervention has been found to be extremely beneficial during traumatic events such as disasters.[10] The basic goals of crisis intervention are to:

- Mitigate the traumatic event's psychological effect
- Facilitate normal recovery processes in those who are having normal reactions to traumatic events

- Restore those affected by the events to a level of functioning commensurate to that before the traumatic event and
- Identify individuals at risk for developing disorders such as PTSD and depression and those in need of more intense counseling.[10]

In addition, 5 key areas of effective crisis planning have been identified, including: (1) planning today for tomorrow's crisis, (2) the ability to respond within 72 hours of an event is crucial, (3) follow-up; (4) being especially vigilant during traumatic event's anniversaries during which some people may experience an increase in distressing memories of the event, and (5) reviewing and reassessing. Effective planning for crisis intervention begins with leadership that can set the policy agenda, secure funds, and bring the necessary people together.[10] Timely and quality planning is crucial to identify, bring together, and manage resources whether internal or external. Those in crisis are more receptive to assistance provided within 72 hours of an event as well as being more motivated to follow through with direction. Individuals and groups at high risk of developing adjustment difficulties should be followed-up, including those who:

- Have acute stress disorder or other clinically significant symptoms stemming from the trauma
- Are bereaved
- Have a preexisting psychiatric disorder
- Require medical or surgical attention and
- Have had a particularly intense and long exposure to the event.[10]

Anniversaries of the event may be particularly traumatic, especially for those experiencing some type of loss. Signs and symptoms may be exhibited as a slight feeling of sadness to a more extensive depression and largely depends on the individual's response to the event as well as coping skills and means of support. Just as timely planning is important, review, and reassessment is of prime importance. Assessing the outcome from emergency and disaster planning as well as incorporating the lessons learned into updated plans of action are fundamental and extremely necessary.

ASSISTING THOSE WITH EXISTING MENTAL HEALTH NEEDS

There are many issues that may be present or that may manifest during a stressful event such as a disaster for those experiencing a disaster and who have established psychiatric or mental health needs.

Medication Management

Medication is an important tool in the treatment and management of those experiencing psychiatric and mental health issues. When not taken on a regular basis and as prescribed, a period of destabilization may transpire, leading to a setback in the treatment and progress. Compounded by the various aspects of a disaster, access to medication can prove to be the most difficult if not impossible task.

In addition, the monitoring of therapeutic medication levels such as levels of drugs in the blood is an important diagnostic tool and should be performed on a routine scheduled basis. Identification of and access to clinical sites that support medication monitoring may be problematic during and after disaster.

Open Communication

Individuals experiencing psychiatric and mental health issues may be experiencing a disruption in thought processes, perceptions, and affects; therefore, establishing and maintaining an open line of communication is necessary. Assisting the individual with an understanding of what has occurred as well as identifying sources of support are key factors to maintaining the stability of the individual. Clarification of thoughts and perceptions may be required on a continuous basis. Providing a safe means to express frustrations or anxieties is also important.

Establishment of Trust

Establishment of trust is a key concept in the patient-provider relationship. During or after a disaster, those most well known to the patient may no longer be available. This unavailability may be a significant loss to the individual, and the situation requires intervention. Therefore, new lines of trust may need to be established and support needs to be provided during the grieving process.

Management of Behavioral Issues

Behavior may be significant in the identification and assessment of a person's response to stress or symptoms of mental disorder or emotional issues. Guidelines for behavior may need to be established, and behavioral or management issues should be addressed during or after a disaster. Delusional thinking or severe anxiety may manifest in an individual, with acting out or negative expression of frustrations or fears demonstrated. Issues with comprehension, reasoning, insight, and judgment may be difficult for an individual undergoing a stressful experience, especially if the experience is prolonged.

Collaborative Efforts

Health care providers play an extremely important role before, during, and after a disaster. However, physical needs may overshadow the psychiatric and mental health needs of those experiencing a disaster. There is a unique opportunity to address the psychiatric and mental health needs by taking a collaborative effort with the community. No person experiencing a disaster is untouched by the experience, and how well a person copes with the experience depends on a multitude of factors, including previous experiences with similar events, the level of life stressors before the event, the effectiveness of coping mechanisms, the actual loss experienced, the level of life stressors before the disaster, and available support systems. Timely and adequate assessment and intervention by health care providers is of key importance. Support systems at the community level such as hospitals, health centers, religious organizations, social organizations, and support groups also play an important role. Schools, churches, and community buildings, such as libraries, are often used as shelters during times of disasters and may provide an optimal setting for the assessment and treatment of those in need of psychiatric and mental health support.

IMPLICATIONS FOR CLINICAL PRACTICE

The psychological effects of disasters are well documented; however, a greater understanding of those with established psychiatric and mental health needs during a disaster is lacking, including a greater understanding of the psychological and psychiatric needs at all levels and age groups during all stages of a disaster. Early intervention is a priority, and an awareness of posttraumatic signs and symptoms is necessary.

Research on the psychological effects and management of disaster is well established, but research on the effects of disasters on those with established psychiatric and mental health needs is limited. A better understanding of how an individual with established psychiatric and mental health issues responds to the stressors during a disaster would provide important information to providers in the preparation and treatment of a vulnerable population.

SUMMARY

Psychological responses to a disaster are well established; however, little is known regarding how individuals with established psychiatric and mental health needs respond to a disaster. Further research is needed to provide a better understanding as well as to provide data and information that would assist in the provision of timely and adequate intervention and treatment. Addressing the psychological and psychiatric needs of this vulnerable population would assist in the provision of adequate and appropriate psychiatric mental health care in a timely and an effective manner.

REFERENCES

1. Inter-American Development Bank. Haiti reconstruction cost may near $14 billion, IDB study shows. Available at: http://www.iadb.org/features-and-web-stories/2010-02/english/haiti-reconstruction-cost-may-near-14-billion-idb-study-shows-6528.html. Accessed May 10, 2010.
2. Centers for Disease Control and Prevention. Disaster mental health primer: key principles, issues and questions. Available at: http//www.bt.cdc.gove/mentalhealth/primer.asp. Accessed May 10, 2010.
3. Kübler-Ross E. On death and dying. New York: Touchstone; 1997.
4. Kessler D. The needs of the dying: a guide for bringing hope, comfort, and love to life's final chapter. Previously published: the rights of the dying. New York: Harper-Collins; 1997.
5. National Alliance on Mental Illness. About mental illness. Available at: http://www.nami.org/Content/NavigationMenu/Inform_Yourself/About_Mental_Illness/About_Mental_Illness.htm. Accessed July 10, 2010.
6. National Institute of Mental Health. Statistics. Available at: http://www.nimh.nih.gov/health/topics/statistics/index.shtml. Accessed July 10, 2010.
7. The United States Department of Health and Human Services, Substance Abuse and Mental Health Services Administration (SAMHSA), National Mental Health Information Center. Homelessness–provision of mental health and substance abuse services. Available at: http://mentalhealth.samhsa.gov/publications/allpubs/homelessness/default.asp. Accessed July 10, 2010.
8. Dosa DM, Hyer K, Brown LM, et al. The controversy inherent in managing frail nursing home residents during complex hurricane emergencies. Controversies in Long-Term Care. J Am Med Dir Assoc 2008;9(8):599–604.
9. Dosa D, Grossman N, Wetle T, et al. To evacuate or not to evacuate: lessons learned from Louisiana Nursing Home administrators following Hurricanes Katrina and Rita. J Am Med Dir Assoc 2007;8:142–9.
10. Prohofsky JA. Preparing for the worst to provide the best response. Behav Health Manag 2005;25(5):12–6.

Catastrophic Events and Older Adults

Elizabeth Cloyd, MBA, RN, NEA-BC[a],*, Carmel B. Dyer, MD[b,c]

KEYWORDS

• Geriatrics • Disasters • Psychosocial needs • Nursing

Inhabitants of every region in the world are susceptible to natural disasters, and for the last several years, the havoc wreaked by hurricanes, tsunamis, and earthquakes on humans has dominated the news. There are 3 general types of disasters that can affect geographic areas. The first type includes disasters that have an immediate or sudden impact, such as bomb detonations, airplane crashes, train accidents, or earthquakes. The second type includes disasters with developing or sustained impact, such as bioterrorism or flu pandemic. The third type includes disasters in which the consequence is such that the essential infrastructure is destroyed, such as the aftermath of a hurricane.[1]

Regardless of the type of disaster, preparedness is the key to saving lives and reducing morbidity and mortality. When Hurricane Rita hit the eastern part of Texas including Houston and surrounding areas in 2005, the city was still recovering from Hurricane Katrina, resulting in an overwhelming reaction to the prospect of another hurricane making landfall on the Gulf Coast. More residents were evacuated than was necessary, resulting in thousands of evacuees spending many hours on gridlocked highways and freeways, where the heat overwhelmed car engines, pets, and in several instances, older persons. In comparison, when Hurricane Ike directly hit Galveston and Houston in 2008, the evacuation of Galveston was started in enough time, while many more Houstonians sheltered in place. Although the effect of the hurricane was devastating to the infrastructure, recovery was much more organized and orderly and the negative impact tempered because of the planning and preparation since 2005.

THE NEED FOR DISASTER PLANNING FOR THE ELDERLY

Despite the fact that older persons comprise 12% of the population and that their numbers will swell to 20% in the next 15 years, before 2005, little planning had focused on meeting their special needs. Older adults are often regarded as having the same capabilities and physiology as other adults; however, much in the same way that neonates differ from children and adolescents, older adults too have unique needs.

The authors have nothing to disclose.
[a] Harris County Hospital District, 2525 Holly Hall, Houston, TX 77054, USA
[b] Geriatric and Palliative Medicine, Lyndon Baines Johnson General Hospital, Houston, TX, USA
[c] University of Texas Health Medical School, Houston, TX, USA
* Corresponding author.
E-mail address: beth_cloyd@hchd.tmc.edu

Crit Care Nurs Clin N Am 22 (2010) 501–513
doi:10.1016/j.ccell.2010.10.003
0899-5885/10/$ – see front matter © 2010 Elsevier Inc. All rights reserved.

Hurricane Katrina highlighted these issues, including the difficulties in providing basic medical care, shelter, and protection from exploitation and abuse. Moreover, compared with younger adults, older adults are more prone to death as a result of natural disasters.[2–4]

Hurricane Katrina uncovered several deficiencies in the approach to the care of older survivors of a natural disaster. About 56% of the evacuees evaluated in the medical unit established in Houston, Texas, by the Harris County Hospital District were 65 years and older. Many of the elderly survivors could not walk to the bathroom or cafeteria, had dementia, and were not aware of their surroundings. Some elderly survivors had sensory impairments that prevented them from reading signs indicating where help was located or hearing the public address system announcements. There were elders who were gravely ill and needed to be hospitalized or moved to a site where their medical needs could be properly addressed.

The need for special planning to accommodate frail elders who required health care services that could not be provided on-site, could not function in an ordinary disaster shelter setting, or could not access the medical services in the shelter because of mental and physical impairments had been overlooked. Some elderly evacuees had friends or family members who assisted them in accessing the wide range of services available in the facility or brought them to on-site medical professionals who arranged for transfer to a more appropriate place, such as a hospital or nursing home. However, many elders had no friends or family and were so debilitated that they could not support themselves or access the on-site services. Usually, they stayed unnoticed as busy volunteers and staff attended to the needs of more able-bodied evacuees.[5] Hurricane Katrina served to underscore the special needs of individuals with disabilities, children, and, especially, unaccompanied older adults.

It has been recommended that every individual, community, and region needs disaster and evacuation plans that address the needs of older adults.[6–8] The assertion that it is vital that nurses be knowledgeable about disaster preparedness and emergency response systems is valid. Nurses should be prepared to teach others about disaster preparedness as well as serve in various roles in community, state, and federal disaster response teams. This article presents the special needs of older adults in disaster situations to help nurses meet the challenges associated with serving this vulnerable population.

GERIATRIC VULNERABILITY

Unlike younger populations wherein grouping according to age is more or less predictable, the older population is extremely heterogeneous. Any given elder might be robust, have chronic illness, or suddenly become frail. Usually, robust elders can provide self-care and protect themselves. Elders with chronic illnesses have greater difficulty in preparing and, if necessary, evacuating. The frail elders may not be able to provide for themselves and require families, friends, or the community to assist them. However, in many instances, both robust elders and those with chronic illnesses rely on physiologic reserves for day-to-day functioning and, when stressed, may not be able to meet the response demands imposed on them by a disaster.[6]

The following section details the physiologic changes that make disaster preparedness, evacuation, and care after the event much more difficult for the elderly. This discussion does not outline all the physiologic changes that occur with aging, but includes cognition, mental capacity and executive function, and functional impairment and also addresses transportation needs as well as susceptibility to exploitation and abuse.

Cognition

The central nervous system is prone to marked changes with aging. Dementia, depression, and delirium are the most common central nervous system disorders that affect older persons.

Dementia

Dementia is a progressive disorder characterized by problems with memory and thinking. Many elders may not recognize early memory changes, and family members and friends often forgive small lapses, assuming they are normal age-related changes. It has been estimated that more than 4 million people in the United States have dementia. This number increases to 26.6 million when the worldwide incidence is considered; nearly 50% of persons older than 85 years have dementia.

Memory loss is the most pervasive symptom of dementia. Some individuals begin to forget names of people they have known all their lives or get lost in familiar places. Because of the nature of the disease, persons with dementia may not remember to pack necessary effects, including their medications. They may become disoriented in an unfamiliar setting such as a shelter. New behavioral problems may arise or otherwise-controlled behaviors may be exacerbated. Several medications are available for the treatment of dementia. The most commonly used medications include acetyl cholinesterase inhibitors and N-methyl-D-aspartate inhibitors. Missed doses of dementia medications can cause a rapid deterioration in function.

Depression

Depression is a mood disorder characterized by withdrawal, lack of energy, and feelings of poor self-worth. Many older persons may not recognize depression or are ashamed of the diagnosis. Depression is seen in about 12% to 15% of older persons in the community, 25% of nursing home residents, 30% of older persons with dementia and Parkinson disease, and nearly 50% of older persons with medical illnesses. The true prevalence may be much higher in older persons because many do not want to admit to a mental illness or screening does not take place. Although age is a risk factor for depression, medical diseases, such as diabetes or renal failure, are more commonly associated with depression.

With the emergence of several selective serotonin reuptake inhibitors, symptoms of depression can be effectively reversed in older persons. Untreated depression can result in cognitive impairment, and an elder with depression can appear to have dementia. Because of the trauma and stress of a natural disaster coupled with depression, the older patients may not be able to effectively extricate themselves or easily negotiate new situations.

Delirium

This disorder is an acute state of confusion, characterized by the inability to attend to tasks and a misperception of reality. Delirium is most commonly seen in older persons after surgery or is associated with acute medical illness. When associated with medical illness, delirium is an emergency. The highest prevalence of delirium (22%–89%) is in persons with dementia.[9] Persons who are delirious are often not aware of the date, where they are, or their circumstances. They may be delusional, have altered sleep-wake cycles, and have garbled or disorganized speech. Health professionals often miss delirium or mistake it for a dementing illness.

Delirium must be detected in disaster situations because it is a risk factor for death.[10] Cases can be easily detected by the Confusion Assessment Method. This tool was developed by Inouye in the 1980s and has been well studied, is sensitive

(94%) and specific (89%), and has even been adapted for the intensive care unit by Ely and Inouye.[11] This tool can help health care professionals to detect delirium and triage older persons to a medical setting where an evaluation of the underlying cause can be done. The most common causes of delirium include infections, medications, electrolyte or blood sugar disturbances, hypoxemia or low oxygen state, and low blood pressure.

Mental Capacity and Executive Function

Mental capacity is defined as the ability to make rational choices and act on them. Decisional capacity refers to the ability to exercise good judgment in determining a course of action. A second component of capacity is executive function, which is the ability to use intention to guide one's actions.[12] Several disorders that plague older persons lead to impaired capacity, including cerebrovascular disease, dementia, depression, malnutrition, psychosis, and substance abuse. At times, older persons who lack decisional and executive capacity may unintentionally put themselves in harm's way. In contrast, a person with capacity has the prerogative to make unwise or unsafe choices.

It is the lack of capacity, particularly executive dysfunction, that makes elders more susceptible to problems during disasters. They lack the ability to plan, sequence, and carry out tasks. The impairment makes disaster preparedness and evacuation difficult for some elders. Assessing capacity is complex; however, 5 instruments have been used when a quick capacity assessment is needed before an operation or procedure, and more are in development (**Table 1**).

Functional Impairment: Mobility and the Senses

In younger individuals, performance and mobility are taken for granted; however, restriction of either can lead to a decline in well-being and result in significant comorbidity. Immobility can result in deconditioning, falls, pressure ulcers, and significant loss of muscle mass. Older persons and their families often assume that the loss of function is a normal part of aging and cannot be reversed. They attribute sedentary tendencies to old age and easily become resigned to inactivity and lower expectations. At times, the loss of function is so gradual that neither the family members nor the affected older persons recognize the changes. Intact functional ability allows an individual to pursue work and leisure activities as well as tackle the stress and injury often associated with disasters. Once function is impaired, individuals are more prone to illness, hospitalization, and the need to move from a residential setting to alternative living situations.

The nurse who assesses a patient in a disaster situation needs to determine how well the patient performs both basic and complex tasks. These tasks include basic activities of daily living (ADLs), such as bathing, toileting, eating, dressing, walking,

Table 1 Quick capacity assessment tools	
Instrument	Authors, Year
Assessing Capacity for Everyday Decisions Instrument	Lai and Karlawish[30], 2007
Capacity to Consent to Treatment Instrument	Marson et al[31], 1995
Executive Interview	Royall et al[32], 2005
Hopemont Capacity Assessment Interview	Edelstein[33], 1999
MacArthur Competence Assessment Tool for Treatment	Applebaum and Grisso[34], 2001

and transferring.[13] More complex tasks are considered as instrumental ADLs (IADLs) and include transportation, administration of medication, cleaning clothes and house-cleaning, use of the telephone, shopping, and cooking. Standard assessments require that older adults make a subjective assessment of their ability to perform ADLs and IADLs. There are several validated, objective, functional assessment tests, such as the Physical Performance Test, which is a timed test of a series of simple tasks.[14]

Vision and Hearing

Older persons experience multiple eye problems with aging. They are prone to several diseases of the lids, lashes, and the eye. Glaucoma is seen in persons older than 40 years, and macular degeneration is the leading cause of blindness in old age. Visual impairment can hamper older persons during disaster situations when relief workers often rely on signs to communicate with large numbers of people. Older adults appreciate large block printing with clear separation of the words when communicating in print. Presbycusis, which makes a person less able to hear high-pitched tones and filter background noise, starts around the age of 50 years. Older persons often misplace hearing aids or its batteries run low, therefore, they are unable to hear instructions given in noisy situations. When communicating with an elder, speaking slowly with monosyllabic words at normal volumes and in quiet settings enhances their comprehension.

Limited Transportation Options

Road safety analysts predict that by 2030, when all baby boomers are at least 65 years old, they will be responsible for 25% of all fatal crashes. According to the National Highway Traffic Safety Administration, drivers older than 65 years are almost twice as likely to die in car crashes as those aged 55 to 64 years.[15] As a result, more groups and states have begun to examine the driving abilities of older adults, both for their own safety and for the safety of others. The American Medical Association asserts that physicians have a responsibility to recognize and document mental and physical impairments that may affect patients' driving safety and pose a risk to the public.[16] Both Florida and Texas have increased requirements for older residents obtaining driving licenses. Florida's requirement that drivers 80 years and older pass a vision test resulted in the loss of driving licenses for about 7% of elderly drivers seeking renewal.[17] The American Association of Neurology recommends any person diagnosed with dementia to stop driving.[18]

All of these restrictions enforced for public safety do limit the evacuation options for older persons. They may think that they cannot rely on help from neighbors or friends who are also evacuating. Public transportation options may be limited in certain regions, overwhelmed by demand, or nonfunctional during a disaster. Families with older members must plan ahead for the needs of those who cannot drive. Communities must also plan for early evacuation of those who cannot drive or who have mobility impairments.

Susceptibility to Exploitation and Abuse

Elder mistreatment (EM) is an international problem and affects persons from all ethnic, cultural, and socioeconomic groups. In 2002, the World Health Organization declared EM to be a worldwide problem.[19] EM is generally considered to include 3 broad types: abuse, neglect, and exploitation. Elder abuse is defined as the infliction of physical harm on a senior and includes sexual assault. Neglect is the failure to provide the goods or services needed to meet basic needs (food, shelter, and medical care). Exploitation is use of an older adult's money or resources by caregivers for their own purposes.[20]

As people age, a variety of biologic changes caused by aging or disease states render them less able to care for and protect themselves. As the need for social and medical support from others increases, so does the risk for EM. A study conducted in 1998 found that elders unable to care for themselves were at a greater risk for abuse, with approximately 60% of elders with substantiated EM experiencing some degree of mental impairment.[21] Experts have estimated that only 20% of EM cases are reported, so EM remains a largely hidden problem. Research has shown that elders who are reported to Adult Protective Services (APS) for physical abuse or caregiver neglect have a mortality rate that is 3 times that of elders never reported to APS.[22] Older adults are more vulnerable during disasters, and displacement caused by evacuation amplifies this vulnerability.

Care for older persons in disasters requires an enhanced sensitivity to exploitation. For example, during Hurricane Katrina, there was exploitation by proprietary owners of nursing homes, apartment landlords, and individuals. Nurses who provide direct care or supervise organizations that serve disaster survivors must carefully screen those who come to assist the elderly, distinguishing them from those who try to take advantage of older adults who are often trusting and may not recognize the unlawful or unscrupulous intentions of others.

VICTIM CONSIDERATIONS

Older adults are more prone to death during a natural disaster. Of the 38 people who died during evacuation from New Orleans to Houston in 2005, the Harris County Medical Examiner's Office noted that 64% (23 of 36 cases) were older than 60 years. All but 4 were classified as natural deaths. Other deaths were classified as suicide (2), accidental (1), and homicide (1). It was later determined that more than 1000 people died in New Orleans, and of those who perished, more than 75% were older adults.[5]

The deaths associated with Hurricane Rita included more accidents. The Medical Examiner's Office identified 45 cases related to the events surrounding the hurricane evacuation. Of the deaths, in 64% (29 of 45) of cases, the decedents were older than 60 years. Seven of the cases were found to be accidental, caused by hyperthermia, and 4 of the decedents were older than 60 years. Most of the deaths were classified as natural, caused by chronic medical problems that were probably exacerbated by the evacuation process.[5] Older adults have more difficulty in evacuating because of physical and cognitive impairments and experience higher mortality rates than younger and more able-bodied evacuees. This observation prompted the following recommendations by members of the Seniors Without Families Triage team (SWiFT) that was formed in Houston during Hurricane Katrina. The SWiFT Tool is a rapid assessment instrument that was administered by a dyad comprising a nurse and a social worker.[5] The following recommendations are adapted from the monograph developed by that team.

Recommendations for Best Practices in the Management of Elderly Disaster Survivors

Develop a simple, inexpensive, cohesive, integrated, and efficient federal tracking system for elders and other vulnerable adults

After Hurricane Katrina, the chairman of the Senate Committee on Health, Education, Labor, and Pensions published a report in which several family members recounted the agony and fear they faced regarding the whereabouts of their frail family members.[5] To safely manage the evacuees, shelter occupants need to be registered. Registration allows central command to track the number of older adults with special needs and devise a strategy to ensure that on-site medical and social services are accessible and available to them.

It may not always be possible for every evacuee to be registered on entry. Some elders may be confused, traumatized, or noncooperative. Those who cannot or do not want to be registered at the time of arrival can be marked with color-coded wrist-bands and identified as unregistered elders. In addition, color-coded wristbands can be used to indicate which elders have been successfully registered, screened, and identified as having special medical or dietary requirements or needing social services.

Use of technology, such as computer-based tracking or electronic cards, in shelter settings has been discussed. Careful consideration should be taken before using this strategy for the geriatric population. Many frail elderly persons who had difficulty in evacuating were impoverished and/or cognitively impaired; therefore, many could not have accessed electronic means for tracking had such means been available before Hurricane Katrina. SWiFT leadership recommended simple and inexpensive color-coded bands. Although there is probably no one-size-fits-all solution, electronic tracking may work in some cases.

Designate separate shelter areas for elders and other vulnerable adults

Shelters should be able to meet the basic needs of special populations, including accessibility to bathing, toilet facilities, and food services. A separate area for the frail elderly and vulnerable adult evacuees should be designated. This demarcation permits easier access by professionals who serve the aging community. In Houston during the Katrina evacuation, able-bodied seniors spontaneously cordoned off an area for themselves and frail elders. Triage to these distinct areas can be accomplished at the time of registration at the facility. When possible, this area should be further divided into separate sections for men and women, taking care not to separate couples or families.

Involve gerontologists (geriatricians, geriatric nurse practitioners, gerontological social workers, or other aging experts) in all aspects of emergency preparedness and care delivery

Many older adults evacuated to the shelter facility with geriatric syndromes, including dementia, psychosis, and delirium, were not identified as needing care at the Katrina Medical Clinic. These adults were not able to self-identify their needs or access help, manage their medications, or obtain meals. These are disorders that are commonly managed by geriatric care teams, and although volunteer health professionals from other disciplines can be helpful in performing triage, the subtleties of these diagnoses could easily elude those not trained in geriatric care. A specialized geriatric medicine unit was formed in the Katrina Medical Clinic and staffed by local geriatricians. In the future, such teams could be located in or near the area where elders and other vulnerable adults are congregated and serve both triage and treatment functions.

Involve region-specific social services, medical and public health resources, volunteers, and facilities in pre-event planning for elders and vulnerable adults

In many instances during a disaster, social needs may be more important than medical needs. Finding housing, ensuring evacuees receive existing benefits, and obtaining disaster relief are critical to their material well-being and mental and physical health. Living day-to-day in a shelter without any plans for return to a more normal setting is extremely disturbing to frail elders who would want to preserve their prior level of independence. Therefore, response teams to the elderly must begin to address social issues as quickly as they address medical issues. Gerontological social workers or nurse case managers with a working knowledge of housing resources, benefit programs, and disaster aid programs are necessary to resolve the nonmedical problems of the frail elders. They must advocate for acquiring the services that evacuees require and for keeping evacuees informed about the progress being made in resolving their problems.

Involve gerontologists (geriatricians, geriatric nurse practitioners, gerontological social workers, or other aging experts) in the training and education of frontline workers and other first responders about frail adults' unique needs
Based on a review of the literature and consultation with experts from the United States, it is unlikely that gerontological nurses participated in disaster planning teams. Had the nurses participated, some of the problems experienced with Hurricane Katrina evacuees might have been avoided. Gerontological nurses have extensive clinical experience with this population; therefore, they should be included in disaster management teams (DMATs) at the federal, state, and local levels. There is a shortage of gerontological health professionals nationally, and at the current enrollment in training programs, there will not be enough professionals to serve on teams in many locales. Gerontological nurses should be encouraged to become part of the DMATs.

Provide protection from abuse and fraud to elders and other vulnerable adults
Decreased cognitive function and physical strength place the elders at risk of exploitation. In the Katrina Medical Clinic in Houston, medications, pocket money, and the few belongings that evacuees still possessed were stolen. Many older adults were exploited for their Federal Emergency Management Agency payments. Operators of residential facilities, many of which were unlicensed, searched the complex for potential business, sometimes moving frail elders who lacked mental capacity to off-site housing facilities. In some cases, the operators took the elders' money and on discovery of the extent of the elders' needs, returned them to the shelter. In shelter situations, it is often difficult to secure the building. The rapid pace involved in trying to move seniors to appropriate living spaces made it difficult to check the quality of every personal care home or senior living center, which resulted in some seniors being placed in apartment complexes when they needed more assistance and supervision than was available.

Utilize a public health triage system for elders and other vulnerable populations in pre-and postdisaster situations
Multiple gerontological professionals from the Houston area volunteered at the Katrina Medical Clinic. These professionals included nurses, social workers, and geriatricians from the Harris County Hospital District and protective service workers from the Texas Department of Family and Protective Services. They noted that family members and friends of frail elders and other vulnerable adult evacuees without family members had no advocates. Therefore, about 8 individuals who serve the elder community in Houston met to devise ways to quickly serve these special-needs populations. It was determined that a rapid screening or triage instrument was needed to determine who needed help, how quickly it was needed, and what interventions could be provided. A tool was devised called SWiFT. The purpose of choosing seniors without family members was to avoid separating families.

Three SWiFT levels were assigned. SWiFT level 1 identified those who needed assistance to perform ADLs, such as bathing, toileting, and remembering to take medications. These persons were to be placed immediately in a more suitable environment, such as a nursing home, a personal care home, or an assisted living facility. SWiFT level 2 identified those with impairments in IADLs who needed assistance to access benefits or manage money. Field team social workers did what they could on the spot and worked on the necessary issues in the ensuing days or referred the evacuees to one of Houston's social service agencies. Persons who were classified as SWiFT level 3 simply needed to be connected to family or had a problem easily remediable by the Red Cross organization or other volunteers.[5] Once the SWiFT tool was piloted and revisions were made, the SWiFT system was put into place.

The SWiFT field teams began by walking through the shelter areas, engaging seniors in conversation. The SWiFT dyads (nurse and social worker) talked to the individual or older couple, asked the questions outlined on the assessment instrument, and filled out the assessment form. During the visit, the nurse would also perform assessments, including that for vital signs. Persons with immediate medical needs were sent for treatment. After a pilot period of 2 hours, the SWiFT teams met again to discuss the effectiveness of the assessment instrument. Modifications were made, and the new assessment instrument was finalized.

Disaster preparedness is key
The SWiFT tool worked well on-site at the Katrina Medical Clinic, and its adoption across Texas proved its utility. This type of triage system is necessary to screen the very sick and the very frail. The SWiFT tool creates a universal language to communicate across jurisdictions. The SWiFT tool and the processes could be adapted for different situations in various regions. It is also important to identify older adults with serious life-limiting diseases, such as metastatic cancer, before the disaster so that palliative care needs are addressed proactively.

All seniors should have a disaster preparedness kit available for immediate evacuation (**Box 1**). A lavaliere wallet, such as that used for airport travel, which is worn around the neck and is waterproof, is ideal for carrying this critical information. Nurses working in primary care, home and public health, nursing facilities, and other senior housing can distribute this list and help older adults be prepared for future events. Restocking the kit and updating information should be done regularly, preferably at the same time each year, for example, on the New Year or on one's birthday.

DISASTER NURSING

Throughout history, nurses have been at the forefront of health care, serving the needs of survivors of disaster. The very origins of nursing are rooted in the care of disaster survivors. The founder of modern nursing, Florence Nightingale, along with her team of nurses, provided care to soldiers of the Crimean War, during which the commitment to care, provide comfort, and use quality practices as recognized at that time saved lives.[23] Later, nurse Clara Barton organized volunteer nurses to become part of the American Red Cross, and at the turn of the twentieth century, nursing became an important component of American Red Cross services. Nurses have been critical members of military health

---

Box 1
Modified Red Cross disaster kit for older adults

Picture identification, social security, and driver's license

Names and phone numbers of relatives and significant others

List of medications with doses and frequency, allergies, and medical diagnoses

Health care information from the physician's office, especially if an electronic medical record is used; health care insurance; and serial numbers and the make of medical devices

Medications for at least 72 hours, kept in original bottles if possible

Hearing aid and wheelchair batteries

care teams since World War II and were part of the mobile army surgical hospital units in Korea, which were the beginning of trauma-response teams.[24,25]

Nurses have been key members of trauma teams since the 1970s when the Emergency Department Nurses Association was established. This organization later became the Emergency Nurses Association, which has included training and certification for disaster survivors. International disaster-response teams, such as the International Committee of the Red Cross and the International Rescue Committee, have acknowledged nurses as integral to their efforts.[25]

ETHICAL CONSIDERATIONS

The 5 principles of ethical considerations in disaster include (1) duty to care, (2) duty to steward resources, (3) duty to plan, (4) distributive justice, and (5) transparency.[26] As organizations develop disaster plans, ethical principles should be followed. In standard mass casualty events, decisions are often made relevant to the survival of the fittest. If advance discussion or planning is not complete, the frail elderly population may disproportionately be left behind. Nurses play a pivotal role in leading discussions and planning disaster response. In the hospital setting, ethics committees should work with disaster committees to consider preparations that could be completed in advance to facilitate the evacuation of the elderly, including considerations for handling immobile patients, managing advance directives and resuscitation orders, and preparing for patients receiving palliative care. Developing a plan prevents hasty or subjective decision making, ensuring that actions taken are collaborative and thoughtful.

NURSING CONSIDERATIONS

Nurses working in the primary care or community health arenas should have extensive plans for education about disaster preparedness. At least once a year, nurses should review and update key information from patients, including the following:

- Changes to living situation
- Ability to perform ADLs
- Availability of caregiver support
- Transportation needs
- Evacuation plans.

In many communities, the city or county may have an evacuation system available for individuals who do not have the means to leave should there be an impending disaster. Ensuring that the elderly in need of this assistance are registered is critical. It behooves any team that is responsible for decisions concerning elders to include nurses and other members who have gerontological experience. The strength of the SWiFT team was that it included community leaders from key organizations as well as gerontological nurses, social workers, and physicians.

CARING FOR THE CAREGIVER: POSTTRAUMATIC STRESS DISORDER AND VICARIOUS TRAUMATIZATION

There is extensive literature concerning posttraumatic stress disorder not only in survivors but also in those who care for the them. Signs and symptoms of posttraumatic stress include

- Subjective and objective components of exposure to trauma
- Reexperience of the trauma

- Persistent avoidance of the trauma or discussion about the trauma
- Increased arousal
- Duration of stress for more than 1 month
- Disturbances causing social and vocational impairment.

Vicarious traumatization is a form of posttraumatic stress disorder. Members of health care rescue teams who are working closely with survivors of disasters often experience vicarious traumatization. They become engrossed in their lifesaving work during the event but may afterward experience psychological distress as a result of their work during the catastrophic event. Vicarious traumatization has been called empathic strain, secondary victimization, or compassion fatigue, and its symptoms include

- Thoughts of the affected people
- Flashes of images of the affected people
- Nightmares
- Hypervigilance
- Avoidance
- Preoccupation with the trauma.[27,28]

It is imperative that disaster responders, emergency workers, and crisis counselors know that they will be affected by the event in some way. Nurses and other health care professionals are cautioned to recognize that they are vulnerable to trauma exposure and should be attuned to the signs and symptoms of these 2 disorders. Nurses must address their own needs to cope with posttraumatic stress disorder and vicarious traumatization and should be prepared to seek professional help from psychologists and psychiatrists.[29]

SUMMARY

The plight of older adults during catastrophic events is a societal concern. Older persons have an increased prevalence of cognitive disorders, chronic illnesses, and mobility problems that limit their ability to cope. These disorders may result in a lack of mental capacity and the ability to discern when they should evacuate or resolve problems encountered during a catastrophe. Some older persons may have limited transportation options, and many of the elderly survivors are at increased risk for abuse, neglect, and exploitation.

Recommendations for future catastrophic events include the development of a federal tracking system for elders and other vulnerable adults, the designation of separate shelter areas for elders and other vulnerable adults, and involvement of gerontological professionals in all aspects of emergency preparedness and care delivery, including training of frontline workers.

Preparation through preevent planning that includes region-specific social services, medical and public health resources, volunteers, and facilities for elders and vulnerable adults is critical. Elders need to be protected from abuse and fraud during catastrophic events. A public health triage system for elders and other vulnerable populations in pre- and postdisaster situations is useful, and disaster preparedness is paramount.

Communities and members of safety and rescue teams must address ethical issues before an event. When older adults are involved, consideration needs to be given to triage decision making, transporting those who are immobile, the care of older adults who receive palliative care, and the equitable distribution of resources.

Nurses are perfectly equipped with the skills, knowledge, and training needed to plan and implement disaster preparedness programs. In keeping with the tradition of Florence Nightingale, nurses can assume several crucial roles in disaster preparedness for older adults. Nurses possess the ability to participate and lead community policy development, serve on rescue teams, perform patient assessments, and deliver care. Nurses are crucial to well-planned and executed programs for catastrophic events that affect older adults. Also, all health care providers involved must be aware of the physical and psychological ramifications of disaster relief. The health and resilience of disaster-relief teams depend on paying attention to signs and symptoms of posttraumatic stress disorder and seeking appropriate treatment should it occur.

REFERENCES

1. Agency for Healthcare Research and Quality (AHRQ). Mass medical care with scarce resources: a community planning guide. Available at: http://www.ahrq.gov/research/mce/mceguide.pdf. Accessed October 6, 2010.
2. Dyer C. Caring for seniors in a national emergency: can we do better? Testimony before the Senate Special Committee on Aging. Washington, DC, May 18, 2006.
3. Cagney KA, Browning CR, Wen M. Racial disparities in self-rated health at older ages: what difference does the neighborhood make? J Gerontol B Psychol Sci Soc Sci 2005;60(4):S181–90.
4. Tanida N. What happened to elderly people in the great Hanshin earthquake? BMJ 1996;313(7065):1133–5.
5. Baylor College of Medicine. Recommendations for best practices in the management of elderly disaster victims. Available at: http://www.bcm.edu/pdf/bestpractices.pdf. Accessed October 6, 2010.
6. Lach H, Langan J, James D. Disaster planning: are gerontological nurses prepared? J Gerontol Nurs 2005;31:21–7.
7. Pekovic V, Seff L, Rothman MB. Planning for and responding to special needs of elders in natural disasters. Generations 2007;31:37–41.
8. Centers for Disease Control and Prevention. The Healthy Brain Initiative: a national public health road map to maintaining cognitive health. Chicago: Alzheimer's Association; 2007. Available at: http://www.cdc.gov/aging/healthybrain/roadmap.htm. Accessed October 6, 2010.
9. Fick DM, Agostini JV, Inouye SK. Delirium superimposed on dementia: a systematic review. J Am Geriatr Soc 2002;50(10):1723–32.
10. Soiza RL, Leslie SJ, Harrild K, et al. Age dependent differences in presentation, risk factor profile, and outcome of suspected acute coronary syndrome. J Am Geriatr Soc 2005;53(11):1961–5.
11. Wei L, Fearing MA, Sternberg EJ, et al. The confusion assessment method: a systematic review of current usage. J Am Geriatr Soc 2008;56(5):823–30.
12. Grimes A, McCullough LB, Kunik ME, et al. Informed consent and neuroanatomic correlates of intentionality and voluntariness among psychiatric patients. Psychiatr Serv 2001;51(12):1561–7.
13. Katx S, Akpom CA. Index of ADL. Med Care 1976;14(Suppl 5):116–8.
14. Reuben DB, Siu AL. An objective measure of physical function of elderly outpatients: the Physical Performance Test. J Am Geriatr Soc 1990;38(10):1105–12.
15. National Highway Traffic Safety Administration. Turning the corner and still driving. Available at: http://www.nhtsa.gov/people/injury/olddrive/TurnThecornerWeb/pages/1background.htm. Accessed October 6, 2010.

16. American Medical Association. Physician's guide to assessing and counseling older drivers. Available at: http://www.ama-assn.org/ama/pub/news/news/older-driver-safety.shtml. Accessed October 6, 2010.

17. Insurance Institute for Highway Safety. Licensing renewal provisions for older drivers. Available at: http://www.iihs.org/laws/olderdrivers.aspx. Accessed October 6, 2010.

18. Dubinsky RM, Stein AC, Lyons K. Practice parameter: risk of driving and Alzheimer's disease. Report of the Quality Standards Subcommittee of the American Academy of Neurology. Neurology 2000;54:2205–11.

19. World Health Organization. World report on violence and health: summary. Available at: http://www.who.int/violence_injury_prevention/violence/world_report/en/summary_en.pdf. Accessed October 6, 2010.

20. US Department of Health and Human Services. The National Elder Abuse Incidence Study. Available at: http://www.aoa.gov/AoARoot/AoA_Programs/Elder_Rights/Elder_Abuse/docs/ABuseReport_Full.pdf. Accessed October 6, 2010.

21. Center of Excellence on Elder Abuse. Elder abuse fact sheet. Available at: http://www.centeronelderabuse.org/files/ElderAbuse_FactSheet_National.doc. Accessed October 6, 2010.

22. Lach MS, Williams CS, O'Brien S, et al. The mortality of elder mistreatment. JAMA 1998;280(5):428–32.

23. Gebbie KM, Valas J, Merril J, et al. Role of exercises and drills in the evaluation of public health in emergency response. Prehosp Disaster Med 2006;21(3):173–82.

24. King B, Jaoti L. Mobile army surgical hospitals: a military and surgical legacy. J Natl Med Assoc 2005;97(5):648–56.

25. Gebbie K, Qureshi K. A historical challenge: nurses and emergencies. Online J Issues Nurs 2006;11(3):2.

26. American Geriatrics Society. Ethical issues in disaster planning: a geriatrics perspective. Available at: http://www.americangeriatrics.org/files/documents/annual_meeting/2010/handouts/wednesday/looking/W0100P_H_Lipman.pdf. Accessed October 6, 2010.

27. Wilson J, Lindy J, editors. Counter-transference processes in the study and treatment of post-traumatic stress disorder. New York: Guilford Press, Inc; 1994.

28. Figley CR. Compassion fatigue. New York: Brunner/Mazel; 1995. p. 5–30.

29. 20th Annual Convening of Crisis Intervention. Vicarious trauma: bearing witness to another's trauma. Available at: http://www.uic.edu/orgs/convening/vicariou.htm. Accessed October 6, 2010.

30. Lai JM, Karlawish J. Assessing the capacity to make everyday decisions: a guide for clinicians and an agenda for future research. Am J Geriatr Psychiatry 2007;15(2):101–11.

31. Marson DC, Ingram KK, Cody HA, et al. Assessing the competency of patients with Alzheimer's disease under different legal standards. A prototype instrument. Arch Neurol 1995;5(10):949–54.

32. Royall DR, Chiodo LK, Polk MJ. An empiric approach to level of care determinations: the importance of executive measures. J Gerontol A Biol Sci Med Sci 2005;60(8):1059–64.

33. Edelstein B. Hopemont capacity assessment interview manual and scoring guide. Morgantown (WV): West Virginia University; 1999.

34. Appelbaum PS, Grisso T. MacArthur competence assessment tool for clinical research (MacCAT-CR). Sarasota (FL): Professional Resource Press; 2001.

Cultural, Ethical, and Spiritual Implications of Natural Disasters from the Survivors' Perspective

Shainy B. Varghese, PhD, RN, CPNP

KEYWORDS

- Survivor • Disaster • Tsunami • Relief

A disaster is defined as an unforeseen event that causes great damage, destruction, and human suffering, which in turn overwhelms the response capacity of local communities, oftentimes necessitating external requests for assistance on a national or international level.[1] These sudden calamitous events that bring about great damage, loss, or destruction can be classified into 2 broad categories: natural disasters and human-made disasters.[2] It seems clear that since the beginning of time, human lives have been disrupted by disasters. It is equally clear that despite the frequently heroic attempts to mitigate the impact of a catastrophic event on a community, a country, or a nation, the effect of a natural disaster has untold consequences for the environment and society.

Advances in technology allow instantaneous communication of the effects of a natural or human-made catastrophe, which has brought increased awareness of the frequency and the profound destruction that may accompany such occurrences. Natural disasters within recent memory include the Indian Ocean tsunami, the Pakistani earthquake, the Kobe earthquake, and Hurricanes Katrina, Rita, and Ike. Within the past year, earthquakes in Haiti and Chile and floods in Pakistan have added to worldwide devastation caused by naturally occurring events. Recent human-made disasters include the terrorist attacks on the World Trade Center, the Gulf oil spill, and the mining accident in Chile.

Annually, millions of people around the world are affected by disasters, and disaster survivors are faced with wide-ranging, often life-threatening dangers, which include large numbers of fatalities; severe injuries; and loss of loved ones, property,

The author has nothing to disclose.

School of Nursing, University of Houston Victoria, Sugar Land Campus, 14000 University Boulevard, Office # 347, Sugar Land, Texas 77479, USA

E-mail address: vargheses@uhv.edu

Crit Care Nurs Clin N Am 22 (2010) 515–522

doi:10.1016/j.ccell.2010.09.005

0899-5885/10/$ – see front matter. Published by Elsevier Inc.

ccnursing.theclinics.com

possessions, neighborhoods, and communities. Adding to the distress of these insults are the effects of the loss of communication with family; fatigue and sleep deprivation; hunger; and emotional or physical strain. Natural disasters may obliterate entire villages or even cities in which survivors have lived since birth. Regardless of the nature of the disaster, human lives are negatively affected and profound societal changes may result. Many investigators have explored the nature of, reasons for, and management of disasters; however, there exists a paucity of literature that details disaster from the victims' perspective. Therefore, this article focuses on the cultural, ethical, and spiritual implications of natural disasters from the survivors' perspective.

CULTURAL IMPLICATIONS OF DISASTER

Culture is used to describe beliefs, ritual practices, art forms, ceremonies, and informal practices such as language, food, and routines of daily life.[3] Culture can be perceived as behavioral responses that have been developed and influenced by social, religious, and intellectual manifestations.[4] Alterations to the social structure of a society can result in disturbances to societal beliefs, ritual practices, art forms, and ceremonies. Culture can be defined in numerous ways, such as ethnic origin, religion, and language. Certain regional areas might share a common culture of their own regardless of their ethnic or religious background. Irrespective of a disaster's causes, a disaster seriously disrupts the life and social structure of individuals, groups, and communities, and may affect the cultural development of the affected region.

Physical health risks and injuries sustained as a result of a disaster are generally similar across cultures, although some variance is seen depending on the severity of the disaster and the availability of timely relief aid. Nonetheless, psychological responses to disaster, loss, and surrounding stressors tend to be slightly different among cultures. Overall, posttraumatic stress disorder, depression, and anxiety seem to be the most common reactions to severe crises and disasters; however, manifestations of psychological distress can vary among cultures.[5,6]

The impact of a disaster on a society is closely related to disaster preparedness, and people prepare, respond, and recover from a disaster within the context of their own culture. Certain cultural groups often do not, or because of the lack of technology and/or communication are unable to, heed warnings about impending disasters. As a result, these groups are inadequately prepared for disaster situations. Developed countries tend to prepare for disasters more thoroughly and further in advance in comparison to developing countries, therefore mitigating some of the resultant devastation.

In some cultures, expressions of trauma are forbidden or strongly discouraged. Various cultures may be more emotionally expressive, whereas others may attempt to carry on as if nothing has happened. Some groups may not need to or may be unwilling to accept assistance from outside parties. An example of this is illustrated in the diametrically opposed response to disaster relief following the earthquakes in Haiti and Chile. The preparedness of the infrastructure as well as economic stability allowed Chileans to handle their disaster response almost entirely within the country, whereas the situation in the impoverished country of Haiti overwhelmed internal resources and necessitated a worldwide response.

Values and Beliefs

According to transcultural nursing theory, the value and belief components of culture influence decision making and actions within the culture. Every community has its own support system and unique manner to deal with crisis situations.[7] Generally, local relief personnel in the affected area manage the initial disaster response. However, a sudden disruption of the social system may cause chaos among individuals in the community because their traditional decision-making bodies no longer exist. The disaster affects the community culture while at the same time requires the mechanisms associated with the culture to facilitate recovery.[8]

When local resources are insufficient, outside assistance is required. Multiple organizations, many of which may be foreign in origin, attempt to undertake relief work with good intentions, but their presence may worsen the situation if they lack knowledge about a community's cultural beliefs. Local customs and traditions may be hard for an outsider to understand, especially if the assistance offered is unfamiliar.

Migration

A disaster can be a strong stimulus that forces people to evacuate from the disaster area. Indeed, mass migration to other areas is not uncommon after a disaster occurs. Temporary or permanent relocation has been a traditional response or survival strategy of people confronted with the prospect, impact, or aftermath of a disaster.[9] Relocation to other parts of a city or locality can disrupt the culture or lifestyle of a community. Moreover, disaster may slow cultural development as populations are forced to move their settlements, resulting in the loss of language, traditional food, clothing styles, or societal status.

After the 2004 Indian Ocean tsunami, the people who lived in the disaster area were required to relocate, but many refused to move. People in the coastal area made their livelihood primarily as fishermen; they had their own culture, local slang, dress, and food. The only job they knew was fishing, so in very tangible ways, postdisaster relocation negatively affected the local culture of these people.

Culture and the Environment

Many rural cultures have developed a sustainable relationship with the environment. Asian cultures attribute spiritual value to the land and environment; in fact, many cultures gain a sense of identity from the land. Indigenous people and ethnic minorities have unique cultures, traditions, language, values, and institutions.[10] When peoples' land and way of life no longer exist, entire cultures may disappear as communities are displaced because of disaster. Distinctive cultures are intimately linked to traditional forms of land and resource management. An example is provided by a report that describes how the cultural heritage of the minority Moken people was seriously affected by the Indian Ocean tsunami. The Moken children no longer care about their language and culture; rather, obtaining material belongings has become the dominant objective in their life.[11]

Culture and Grief

Cultural beliefs can function as both a resource and a barrier in providing support for grieving families. A cross-cultural perspective reveals an enormous variety in peoples' responses to death and the ways in which they mourn. Certain cultures have specific rituals that must be followed after death. These rituals help individuals to move from a maladaptive to an adaptive style of grieving. Cultural insensitivity to the grieving process can have a negative psychological effect on the survivors. Therefore, sensitivity to cultural needs for ritual in response to death and providing privacy are crucial to relief responses.

ETHICAL IMPLICATIONS OF DISASTER

Addressing the many ethical issues that are encountered during disaster relief can be perplexing because cultural differences may lead to confusion about right and wrong. Ethical approaches refer to well-founded standards of what humans ought to do in terms of rights, obligations, benefits to society, fairness, or specific virtues.[12] A confounding factor, particularly for first responders is that actions considered ethically right in one area might be considered wrong in other locales. Ethical issues may be seen entirely differently from victims' perspectives as compared with disaster management personnel or observers. From a victim's perspective, the major ethical issues in a disaster are often related to allocation of resources and protecting their privacy and their property.

Conducting a timely and accurate needs assessment is a critical component of appropriate resource allocation. Immediately after a disaster, various relief organizations and agencies begin compiling needs assessments, sometimes without crucial information such as the availability of resources and the ability to provide support. Unless these agencies are in a position to provide assistance to needy people in a timely manner, it is unfair to perform a needs assessment as it may give victims a false hope. For example, one of the survivors of Indonesian tsunami stated that "immediately after the earthquake they said we would receive 30 days of emergency supplies and food; so far we have received only 5 days."[13]

Sustainability of assistance is another problem. If relief agencies arrive in affected areas and provide high-tech solutions for only a few weeks' time, their subsequent departure may only cause more frustration for the victims. When assistance is offered initially, the affected community may not make use of their own resources. When aid is suddenly withdrawn, victims may find themselves in a worse state than if the agency had not come at all, particularly if the solutions are unsustainable. In some instances, it may better serve the community for them to create their own local support system to manage the disaster because uninvited or well-meaning assistance may serve to disrupt existing social systems.

Immediately after the Indian Ocean tsunami, television crews, relief agencies, and rescue personnel inundated affected areas. Bodies were pulled out of rubble, survivors were sent to displacement camps, and thousands of people were made newly homeless. For those who survived the initial catastrophe, the battle to stay alive truly began when the tsunami waters receded.[13] Devastating for the survivors was the fact that as a result of the flooding, their basic living accommodations such as beds, appliances, and furnishings—items they sometimes had saved for years to buy—were unusable. Worse still was not only the annihilation of individual homes, neighborhoods, and communities but also the disruption of the infrastructure, including fresh water and electricity.

Food, clothing, and shelter are basic human needs, and food and dress are major components of a culture. Often after a disaster, relief organizations collect nonperishable food and clothing to send to survivors. Although these items are sent with the best of intentions, their actual usage may depend on how culturally appropriate these things are in the community to which they have been provided.

Barriers to Resource Management and Aid

A large proportion of the aid allocated to an area may never reach the victims. Reasons for this are varied; for example, in developing countries, it is not uncommon for mediators to take advantage of a catastrophic event to reap financial gain from the dire predicament of the survivors. Corruption on a political level and the vested interests of leaders or administrators can create a logjam for resources intended for needy people. Across tsunami-affected areas of India, just 28% of the total 98,447 required houses have been built. In the Andaman and Nicobar Islands where 9147 homes are needed, reconstruction so far is less than 1%.[14] Inequitable allocation of resources is another ethical issue related to resource management.

In Sri Lanka, relief efforts were stymied by political interference, bureaucratic bottle-necks, and ethnic strife, resulting in construction of fewer than half of the required 110,000 houses. Most of the homes that have been built are located in the southern part of Sri Lanka, whereas the east and north of the country remains grossly neglected.[14] There are few publicized examples of allocation mismanagement; many others remain unreported.

Using resources for survival is different from taking nonessential luxury items for profit; however, it is not uncommon in developing countries for looters to travel to disaster sites. Their pretense is to act as if they are helping the community while in reality they are pilfering resources that are badly needed by the survivors. Researchers have studied mass looting after community crises. In 1985, when Hurricane Hugo affected the US Virgin Islands, the scale of city looting initiated by organized gangs of delinquent youths was massive.[15]

Triaging the limited resources that exist in a disaster's aftermath is the most difficult aspect of disaster management. Resources include materials, labor, personnel, and financial assistance. For example, decisions must be made regarding a limited water supply, including whether water should be disseminated in such a way that everyone receives a small, perhaps inadequate, portion or provided so that greater quantities are distributed to a smaller population. The same concept applies in the case of food and shelter—the decisions made constitute another ethical dilemma. In regard to human rights and obligations, the victims might feel that their rights ought to be pro-tected no matter the cost.

PROTECTING THE PRIVACY AND PROPERTY OF VICTIMS

A disaster's aftermath is something that no one wants to remember; however, the media is often intrusive to those who are suffering or mourning over their losses. The loss of loved ones, sometimes entire families, are times for privacy and respect for the deceased, which is disrupted when the media telecast survivors in their stricken and devastated states as they mourn. During the Indian Ocean tsunami, the media televised images of dead bodies floating in the water and corpses that had not been covered properly in morgues. Media coverage of weeping relatives and the deceased was deeply disturbing not only to the victims but also to many viewers. Sometimes filming injured victims after the disaster is used for commercial purposes, such as promoting the program to television stations and newspapers or for charity fund-raising.[16] The infringement on the privacy of those left emotionally shattered is disrespectful not only to the living but also to those who lost their lives.

Different types of media personnel at the same site may overcrowd hospitals and hamper the efficiency of the health care system. The media complicate the task at hand, as their demands divert rescuers' attention from urgent matters such as casu-alty care, search, rescue, and evacuation. Some advantages of the media include a higher level of worldwide attention and receiving necessary help in a timely manner.[17] For example, the involvement of the media in the Indian Ocean tsunami helped a young boy find his relatives.

Disaster Research

Disaster researchers are another group of people who invade the privacy of the victims. Disaster research is important and can be performed concurrently or retrospectively. Nonetheless, the victims often perceive disaster research as emotionally torturing because survivors are asked questions specific to the disaster. Finding loved ones and caring for them is the priority for disaster survivors. Although data collection is necessary to assess the situation, it is often seen as unfair and intrusive to the people who are in distress.

SPIRITUAL IMPLICATIONS

Spirituality defines that area within the self where persons respond to the call of transcendence.[18] In times of distress and need, individuals may look toward their spiritual or religious beliefs to help them cope. The sudden and overwhelming nature of the disaster trauma creates many questions for the victims and the survivors. Some disaster survivors' beliefs may be affected negatively because of the traumatic experience, resulting in questioning of God's existence or even a complete loss of faith.[19]

Some religions believe that disasters are signs of God's wrath, whereas others believe that God allows disasters to occur because of the sinful nature of man. Questions sometimes arise for believers as they struggle, for example, to understand the many children killed in the Asian tsunami and the reason such things happen to innocent children. Despite this struggle, however, many disaster survivors report that their spiritual beliefs strengthened after a catastrophic event. Individuals who survived the September 11, 2001, terrorist attacks on the World Trade Center reported an increase in spirituality, and during Hurricane Katrina, survivors reported that God's image served as a coping mechanism that allowed them to create meaning in their lives and adjust to their disturbing experiences.[20,21] About 50% of the Indian Ocean tsunami survivors claimed that the disaster had strengthened their relationship with God.[22] Catastrophe can also wash away layers of superficiality and enable human beings to relate on a deeper level. For example, it was reported that after 9/11 people focused more on their relationships with their spouse and children.[22]

SUMMARY

Cultural, ethical, and spiritual implications of disaster depend on various factors. The impact of a disaster on a particular culture depends on the people in that culture and the strength and resilience of the culture. Disasters may slow cultural development; however, typically the customs, beliefs, and value systems remain the same even if the outward expressions of culture change. Critical to survivors is the implication of aid that is culturally sensitive.

Ethical questions and dilemmas associated with disasters and their management are profound. Adhering to ethical principles does not solve all of the issues related to disaster management, but awareness of their utility is important. People affected by a disaster may not be capable of responding to human rights violations, so it is the first responders who must be cognizant of their responsibility to protect the victims' dignity and rights.

Ethical treatment of survivors entails a crucial blend of knowledge about ethnic culture, religious beliefs, and human rights. A strong awareness of ethical principles is merely a beginning step to well-informed decision making in disaster situations. The literature also suggests that during a crisis, spirituality helps victims to cope. Important to any catastrophic event is the understanding that every disaster creates unique circumstances that require relief responses tailored to the specific situation.

REFERENCES

1. Center for Research on the Epidemiology of Disasters. Disasters in numbers. Center for Research on the Epidemiology of Disasters. 2006. Available at: http://www.unisdr.org/eng/media-room/press-release/2007/2006-Disaster-in-number-CRED-ISDR.pdf. Accessed May 20, 2010.
2. International Strategy for Disaster Reduction (2006). United Nations strategies for disaster reduction. 2005. Available at: http://www.unbrussels.org/agencies/unisdr.html. Accessed May 20, 2010.
3. Weinreich P. Identity structure analysis. In: Weinereich P, Saunderson W, editors. Analyzing identity: cross cultural, societal and clinical contexts. New York: Routledge; 2003. p. 7–76.
4. Giger JN, Davidhizar RE. Transcultural nursing: assessment and intervention. St Louis (MO): Mosby; 1999.
5. Zhang H, Zhang Y. Psychological consequences of earthquake disaster survivors. Int J Psychol Special issue: The psychological dimensions of global change 1991;26:613–21.
6. Neria Y, Olfson M, Gameroff MJ, et al. The mental health consequences of disaster-related loss: findings from primary care one year after the 9/11 terrorist attacks. Psychiatry 2008;71(4):339–48. Available at: http://www.biomedexperts. com/Abstract.bme/19152283/The_mental_health_consequences_of_disaster-related_loss_findings_from_primary_care_one_year_after_the_9_11_terrorist_at. Accessed April 15, 2010.
7. Leininger M, McFarland MR. Transcultural nursing: concepts, theories, research, and practice. 3rd edition. New York: McGrath-Hill; 2002.
8. Deeny P, McFetridge B. The impact on culture, self, and identity: increased awareness by health care professionals is needed. Nurs Clin North Am 2005; 40(3):431–40.
9. Hugo G. Environmental concerns and international migration. Int Migr Rev 1996; 30(1):105–31.
10. Chino T. Asia Development Bank: speech to the regional workshop on indigenous people and poverty reduction. October 25, 2001. Available at: http://www.adb. org/Documents/Speeches/2001/ms2001073.asp. Accessed April 15, 2010.
11. Nidhiprabha B. Adjustment and recovery in Thailand two years after tsunami. Asia Development Bank Institute; 2007. Available at: http://www.adbi.org/discussion-paper/2007/08/02/2344.thailand.tsunami.adjustment.recovery/. Accessed September 30, 2010.
12. Velasquez M, Andre C, Shanks T, et al. What is ethics? Markkula Center for Applied Ethics; Fall, 1987. Available at: http://www.scu.edu/ethics/practicing/decision/whatisethics.html. Accessed September 30, 2010.
13. Taylor J. What happens in a disaster zone after the news crew go home. Independent World. January 23, 2010. Available at: http://www.independent.co.uk/news/world/.
14. Macan-Marker M. Tsunami recovery hit by corruption, apathy. Inter Press Service News Agency; December 7, 2006. Available at: http://ipsnews.net/news.asp? idnews=35984. Accessed September 30, 2010.
15. Quarantelli K, Frailing K. (2007). Looting after disaster: a myth or reality. Natural Hazard Observer. XXXI 4 March 2007. Available at: http://www.colorado.edu/hazards/o/archives/2007/mar07/index.html. Accessed September 30, 2010.
16. Bhan A. Should health care professional allow reporters inside the hospitals and clinics at the time of natural disasters? PLos Med 2005;2(6). Available at: www. plosmedicine. Accessed September 30, 2010.

17. Auf der Heide E. Disaster response principle of preparation and coordination. 1989. Available at: http://orgmail2.coe-dmha.org/dr/PDF/DisasterResponse.pdf. Accessed September 30, 2010.

18. Parrella FJ. Spirituality in crisis: the search for transcendence in our therapeutic culture. Spirituality today Winter 1983;35(4):292–303. Available at: http://www.spiritualitytoday.org/spir2day/833541parrella.html. Accessed May 25, 2010.

19. Koenig HG. In the wake of disaster: religious responses to terrorism and catastrophe. Philadelphia: Templeton Press; 2006.

20. Peterson C, Seligman MEP. Character strengths before and after September 11. Psychol Sci 2003;14:381–4.

21. Aten JD, Moore M, Denny RM, et al. God images following hurricane Katrina in South Mississippi: an exploration study. J Psychol Theol 2008. Available at: http://www.thefreelibrary.com/. Accessed May 25, 2010.

22. Rigler, S.Y. (January 5, 2005). After disaster. Aish.com Available at: http://www.aish.com/ci/be/48892392.html. Accessed May 29, 2010.

Disaster Aftermath: A First-Person Perspective as a Responder and Caregiver

Michael L. Mistric, PhD, RN, FNP, BC[a,b,]*, Tobin A. Sparling, JD[c]

KEYWORDS

• Mitigation • Preparedness • Response • Recovery

During the period following World War II and at the onset of the "Cold War," the prevailing term used for emergency or disaster management was "Civil Defense." Although civil defense evokes images of air-raid drills and bomb shelters, the system also encompassed strategies to warn about, respond to, and survive impending natural disasters such as hurricanes, tornados, and other severe weather events. As the human responses to disaster received greater scientific study, the term civil defense gave way to the more academic-sounding "disaster management." Today, disaster management "aims to reduce, or avoid, the potential losses from hazards, assure prompt and appropriate assistance to victims of disasters, and achieve rapid and effective recovery" through the coordinated efforts of government, businesses, and civil society.[1]

The experiences and lessons of catastrophic natural events in the 1980s and 1990s, including hurricanes, tornados, and earthquakes, as well as human-made events such as the terrorist attacks of 9/11 led to a focus on the "before-and-after" periods of disaster from the perspective of both the victim and the responder.[2,3] Numerous books and articles describe the phases of disaster management in generalized terms and largely from the victim's perspective. In contrast, this article describes the

---

The authors have nothing to disclose.

The opinions herein are those of the writer, and do not necessarily reflect the views of the Department of Veterans Affairs.

[a] Extended Care Line, Michael E. DeBakey VAMC, 2002 Holcombe Boulevard, Houston, TX 77030, USA

[b] Texas Woman's University, Houston, TX, USA

[c] South Texas College of Law, 1303 San Jacinto Street, Houston, TX 77002, USA

* Corresponding author. Nurse Practitioner–Nu2C, Extended Care Line, Michael E. DeBakey VAMC, 2002 Holcombe Boulevard, Houston, TX 77030.

E-mail address: michael.mistric@va.gov

Crit Care Nurs Clin N Am 22 (2010) 523–534

doi:10.1016/j.ccell.2010.09.004

0899-5885/10/$ – see front matter. Published by Elsevier Inc.

ccnursing.theclinics.com

4 phases of disaster management, including (1) mitigation, (2) preparedness, (3) response, and (4) recovery from the perspective of a health care provider (**Fig. 1**).

Author's note: I serve as a family nurse practitioner at the Michael E. DeBakey VA Medical Center in Houston, Texas (hereafter "Houston VA"). I participated directly in each of the 4 phases of disaster management preparation and response as a member of the Houston VA's patient reception team, which was established to take action during hurricane-related disasters.

I served as a first responder and caregiver in the period leading up to, during, and after Hurricane Katrina. In this article, I recount my experience of each of these phases, and draw lessons from them.

THE MITIGATION PHASE

Mitigation has been described as the cornerstone of emergency management. Defined as "the sustained action that reduces or eliminates the long-term risks to people and property from natural or human-made disasters and their effects,"[2] mitigation occurs before disaster. Mitigation encompasses community activities to prevent a disaster, to reduce the chances of a disaster occurring, and to lessen the damages resulting from disaster.[2]

Following 9/11, President George W. Bush established the US Department of Homeland Security.[4] The National Disaster Medical System (NDMS) was created under the jurisdiction of the US Department of Homeland Security, Federal Emergency Management Agency, Response Division, and Operations Branch.[4,5]

NDMS was chartered to support federal agencies in the management and coordination of the federal medical response to such emergencies as natural disasters, technological disasters, major transportation accidents, and acts of terrorism including

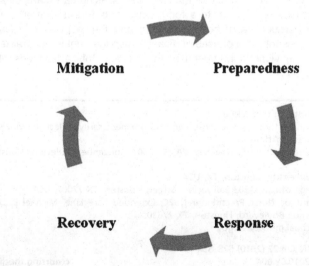

Mitigation   **Preparedness**

Recovery   **Response**

Fig. 1. Disaster management cycle.

weapons of mass destruction events.[5] Designated to "design, develop, and maintain a national capability to deliver quality medical care to the victims of and the responders to a domestic disaster," NDMS provides (1) medical response to a disaster area in the form of teams, supplies, and equipment; (2) patient movement from a disaster site to unaffected areas of the nation; and (3) definitive medical care at participating hospitals in unaffected areas.[5]

Four federal partners of the NDMS have combined their efforts to establish a single national medical response capability to "assist state and local authorities in dealing with the medical and public health effects of major peacetime disasters."[5] The 4 partners are (1) the Department of Health and Human Services, (2) the Federal Emergency Management Agency, (3) the Department of Defense, and (4) the Department of Veterans Affairs.[5]

The Creation of the Patient Reception Team

Spurred by these federal initiatives, the Houston VA began the process of disaster mitigation in 2003 with the creation of a patient reception team. The resulting group of health care professionals and hospital support personnel became known as the Michael E. DeBakey VAMC Patient Reception Team. Although the patient reception team was formulated as part of a national effort, its mission was heavily influenced by a local natural disaster. In 2001, Tropical Storm Allison left many parts of Houston flooded. The Texas Medical Center in Houston was particularly hard hit. Many of its health care providers suffered interruptions of service, in large part because of catastrophic damage to their electrical plants. In light of this experience and owing to Houston's proximity to the Gulf of Mexico, the Houston VA patient reception team determined its primary goal to be the mitigation of damages from hurricanes and similar weather-related emergencies.

Houston VA health care professionals and hospital support personnel were asked to volunteer for the patient reception team. Those interested convened to plan strategies. From the very beginning, it was assumed that people in need of medical care would be airlifted from storm-affected areas. The patient reception team would receive those patients, process them, and coordinate their transport to appropriate medical facilities for further care. The team was led by an operations chief who oversaw its direction and management. As initially conceived, the operations chief would receive the patient manifest; coordinate immediate transport of critically ill patients; liaise with airport personnel, fire department personnel, police, Houston VA personnel, security, and NDMS representatives; and create the staffing plan for the providers assigned to the patient reception team.

The team used Ellington Field, a local National Guard airport, as its staging area. An airplane hangar at the field was designated for the team's practice exercises. To prepare for an actual event, the team made arrangements with the Air National Guard to fly in "volunteer" patients to give realization to the disaster exercises. A decision was made to invite personnel from other medical centers in Houston to join the team, completing the mitigation phase of the patient reception team disaster management plan.

THE PREPAREDNESS PHASE

The second phase of emergency management is preparedness. Preparedness takes the form of plans and/or procedures designed to save lives and minimize damage when an emergency occurs.[2] Planning, training, and disaster drills are the essential elements of preparedness. Although the foundation of preparedness is planning the types of activities that will take place before, during, and immediately after a disaster occurs, it should not be confused with the mitigation phase.[2]

Training and Fine-Tuning the Patient Reception Team

From 2003 through 2005, the patient reception team met twice a year to plan, implement, practice, and refine its operations. Before each practice session, the team reviewed its flow chart and participant responsibilities. After each exercise, debriefing allowed the team to review aspects of the exercise that went well and determine areas for improvement. The importance of this step was obvious as the team grew increasingly proficient with each practice session.

At the first exercise, in 2003, those responsible for medical treatment developed the plan for organizing the flow of disaster victims, determining the best possible patient flow layout. Mock patients supplied by the Air National Guard were used to put the patient flow plan to the test. Following this disaster drill, the team met to further refine its operations. Most importantly, adjustments were made to the staging plan, creating a 4-tiered administrative structure under the command of the operations chief. The respective tiers were led by a transportation manager, a patient access manager, a registered nurse (RN) coordinator, and a patient flow administrator (**Fig. 2**).

The transportation manager was responsible for the movement of each patient from the time the patient was released from the aircraft to the staging area until the patient was released for transport to a medical or evacuation center. Creating a staffing plan and training staff for the transportation section was a key assignment. In addition, the transportation manager coordinated sanitation and waste management services.

The patient access manager created and managed a staffing plan for the patient access section. Responsible for collecting patient information and demographics from check-in to check-out, the patient access manager provided a bed count for all NDMS medical and evacuation facilities, coordinated the transfer from the staging area to the medical and evacuation facilities, and established phone contact with the receiving medical facility before transfer.

The registered nurse coordinator was responsible for the staffing plan for the nurses of the patient reception team. The RN coordinator managed patient flow from the time the patient was logged at the registration station until the patient was taken to the holding area for transport to a medical or evacuation facility. Assisting with the identification of emergent patients for immediate transport, directing patients to the triage holding area and to each of the triage stations for medical evaluation, as well as to a patient waiting area to await post-triage transportation to a medical or evacuation facility were key assignments. Additional tasks included overseeing the team's pharmaceutical and medical supplies in conjunction with a pharmacist and a medical

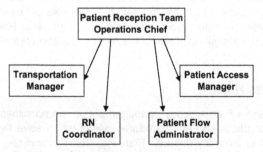

Fig. 2. Patient reception team administrative structure.

supply representative. Finally, the RN coordinator assisted in the identification of individuals needing isolation and managed the isolation area.

The patient flow administrator was a health systems specialist who provided administrative support to the patient reception team by working directly with the operations chief. The patient flow administrator received the patient manifest and provided copies to the appropriate stations. In addition, the patient flow administrator created the staffing plan and schedule and maintained a roster of patient reception team names and contact information had additional resources been required.

The team held another disaster drill at Ellington Field in 2004. The efforts of the previous year's training paid off as evidenced by improved organization. Medical providers further anticipated the types of casualties encountered and reviewed the appropriate care that would need to be provided. Practicing clinical skills was maximized owing to the presence of mock disaster victims simulating a range of general medical, surgical, and psychological conditions.

At this drill, the team realized that as providers with responsibility for being available during a disaster, personal planning to ensure for the safety of families and property was needed. Making arrangements for family, including decisions regarding whether to evacuate, as well as preparation, including such things as reinforcing storm windows, gathering appropriate supplies, and making lists of perishable supplies to be collected in an imminent disaster, were critical steps that ensured that each team member would be ready to respond immediately, without concern about the safety of loved ones or property.

THE RESPONSE PHASE

The third phase of disaster management is the response phase. The response phase includes actions taken to save lives and prevent further damage during and immediately following the disaster or emergency situation.[2] The response phase involves putting preparedness plans into action. The health care provider's role in the response phase includes such activities as rendering emergency medical care at the scene, as well as staffing local health care facilities to provide physical and psychological medical and nursing care.[2,6]

Hurricane Katrina

On August 29, 2005, Hurricane Katrina, a Category 3 hurricane, made landfall over Biloxi, Mississippi. Although New Orleans appeared to have been largely spared, its levees gave way a day later, leaving much of the city deluged. As the city flooded, the health care infrastructure became severely compromised, necessitating the evacuation of the sick and injured out of the city.

The Patient Reception Team Goes into Action

On Monday, August 29, 2005, the operations chief notified the patient reception team that it would be activated. Upon arrival at Ellington Field, the receiving facility was set up as supplies and equipment were unloaded from trucks. (**Fig. 3** illustrates the Patient Reception Team Flow Chart for evacuee processing.) A triage holding area, staffed by a registered nurse was positioned between the check-in station and triage stations. A provider at the check-in station assessed for patients needing immediate emergent transport. Each triage station included a provider (physician, physician assistant, or nurse practitioner), and 2 nurses (registered nurse and licensed vocational nurse and/or nursing assistant). A psychiatrist was available in the triage station area to handle mental health issues of patients and/or staff. Every triage station had

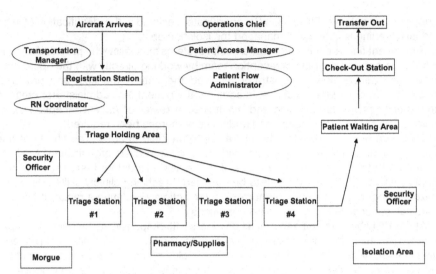

Fig. 3. Patient reception team flow chart.

a stretcher, a supply cart, and vital sign monitoring equipment. The nursing staff ensured that the supply carts had adequate supplies for starting intravenous (IV) lines and providing basic first aid.

Immediately behind the triage station, a pharmacist was posted to dispense medications and ensure that adequate medication and supply levels were maintained. The pharmacist also maintained security of controlled substances. Based on established standards and recommendations, the pharmacist, along with the operations director and the RN coordinator, established medication and supply levels, modifying them to fit the situation. To provide support for evacuees, a chaplain and social worker were stationed in the patient waiting area. The social worker was available to answer or assist with any patient and/or family social needs, whereas the chaplain addressed spiritual needs. Security officers were strategically positioned in the areas between the triage holding area and the triage stations and between the triage stations and the patient waiting area. Thus, officers would be immediately at hand should any security issues arise.

The team had about 2 hours to prepare for the first incoming evacuees. Before staffing the positions on the team flow chart, the team members reviewed their role responsibilities and the patient flow sequence and were updated about available supplies and equipment. The patient reception team operations chief, in collaboration with the transportation manager, lined up all available ambulances to be ready to receive patients. When the first airplane landed, the patient reception team operations chief, the medical director, and the transportation manager reviewed the patient manifest with either the aircraft crew chief or the pilot. At that point, a determination was made regarding whether any patients needed immediate evacuation to a local medical facility or required isolation. Those needing immediate transport were loaded directly onto an ambulance while the patient access manager made arrangements for transfer to a local medical facility for further evaluation and care (**Fig. 4**). Isolation patients were taken to an isolation station at the back of the triage area away from the main patient flow, remaining there until appropriate disposition could be made.

Following these assessments, the transportation manager signaled for stretchers to move patients to the patient reception area. Once assigned to a specific patient, the

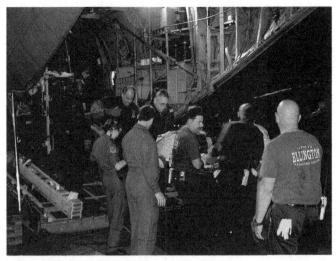

Fig. 4. Evacuated patients arriving at Ellington Field.

Author's note: After I was notified, a flaw in the team's planning immediately became apparent. We had failed to adequately consider how staffing and patient care would be handled in the absence of members of the patient reception team when they were called upon to respond.

I work as a mid-level provider on a 120-bed, long-term care inpatient service divided into four 30-bed units. Each unit is managed by an attending physician and a nurse practitioner or physician assistant. I managed one of those units. I asked providers who were not involved with the patient reception team to volunteer to care for my inpatients. The providers rallied and devised a plan to staff my unit.

In the course of planning, my service anticipated that if evacuees came from New Orleans, we would have to make space for those needing long-term care. We designated my 30-bed unit as the unit for such evacuees. With the help of our department medical director and social workers, my 30 existing patients were temporarily moved to other long-term care units in our facility. Some patients were discharged to home if their families were in the position to care for them for a short period. We discharged patients who had no family members or other support systems in place to community nursing homes willing to accept them under the circumstances.

Two days later, on August 31, 2005, the team received word that the first aircraft with evacuees from New Orleans would arrive at Ellington Field that evening. We immediately went to Ellington Field to set up to receive patients. I contacted my family and let them know where I was going and that I did not know when I would be home. After that, I called my supervisor who notified another nurse practitioner of the need to cover my patients for that day.

transporters remained with that patient throughout the entire process until the patient was placed on an ambulance or other appropriate transportation. The provider working the registration station met each patient to determine the immediacy of the need for transport while a registration station representative obtained identification information. If any patient was determined to be emergent, the patient was diverted directly to transport to the nearest hospital. Following the registration process, patients not needing immediate transport were moved to the triage holding area where

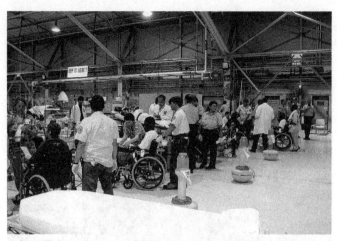

Fig. 5. View of patient reception team Triage Stations at Ellington Field.

a registered nurse coordinator triaged each patient to a specific triage station for further evaluation, ensuring that family units were kept together as much as possible (**Fig. 5**).

The staff at the triage station determined the need for IV therapy, pain medication administration, blood pressure management, and any other immediate medical or nursing requirements. After being assessed and stabilized, patients were tagged with a color-coded identification tag (emergent, immediate, or delayed) to identify the immediacy of their need for transport. The transporters then moved the patient to the patient waiting area to await transfer to a medical facility or refugee evacuation site. After the patient was loaded onto the appropriate vehicle, the patient access management staff noted this information at the check-out station. When all the triage stations were occupied, the registered nurse coordinator managed the remaining patients in the triage holding area until a triage station was free, ensuring that as soon as a station was available, a transporter was notified to bring another patient to the available triage station.

The patients on the first and all subsequent aircraft ran the gamut—adults, children, elderly, and families—all of whom needed to be moved through the system as a unit so they would not be separated. Some patients needed dialysis, others had infected wounds, and many had lost their medications. There were patients from hospitals who had recently had surgery and subsequently were evacuated down multiple flights of stairs in postsurgical status. Within the first few hours, the lack of pediatric supplies and equipment became obvious. Local community hospitals were contacted to provide obstetric, gynecologic, and pediatric services. They sent appropriate staff, equipment, and supplies, including their pediatric crash carts.

Author's note: One of the things we had not anticipated in our drills and preplanning was the need for backup to relieve the initial members of the team at Ellington Field. Because we had no relief schedules, team members had to remain at Ellington Field throughout the first day and night until relief could be arranged.

The Houston VA arranged for food and cots. Between transport arrivals, we slept and ate when we were not cleaning the areas and restocking supplies. Needless to say, by afternoon of the next day, the first responders were tired.

Within the first 24 hours, volunteers from the Houston VA and other facilities in the surrounding community began to arrive to relieve the patient reception team members. Challenges lay in orienting the new staff to the supplies, their assigned roles, and patient flow. The volunteers were eager and dedicated to the mission, and everyone was focused on the evacuees and their needs. As relief workers arrived, the patient reception team director along with the RN coordinator devised a work schedule including the team members and the additional volunteers from the VA and the community, rotating on and off at 8-hour or 12-hour shifts.

Author's note: Although no one knew exactly what to expect once the evacuees arrived, we were prepared for almost anything; however, found that we had not sufficiently anticipated the emotional strains we would face.

I encountered one family—a single mother with 5 children in tow. The oldest was 11 and the youngest was just a few months old. After they came off the transport plane, they were escorted to the hangar. I happened to be the one to take them for evaluation. After finding everyone to be clinically sound, I took the family to meet the social worker who would help them find a place to stay, as they did not need to be hospitalized. The mother stated she had left New Orleans with a few possessions they could carry and the clothes on their backs. She said she had lost everything, but she was trying to keep her family together.

This was a heart-wrenching moment for me. As a clinician, I am able to handle clinical situations that come my way, but this social situation was all I could handle. After I made sure they would be looked after, I talked with the chaplain about how the situation had affected me emotionally. The chaplain assured me this was a normal response for caregivers in a disaster situation. He was there to help the evacuees and the health care providers as both, in different ways, were victims of the disaster.

The mission lasted for 5 days and during that time the patient reception team received and logged in more than 800 patients from 21 flights. After the fifth day, a skeleton staff was available until all evacuations ceased. As operations came to a close, planning for providing care for New Orleans veterans who had been evacuated to Houston began. While still at Ellington Field, the team leadership drafted plans to open a Houston MEDVAMC-based clinic in the hospital gymnasium specifically for these veterans. The clinic, staffed by both New Orleans and Houston VA staff, opened within a week of the end of the mission at Ellington Field. It remained open for about 1 year, after which New Orleans veterans were managed in the Houston VA outpatient clinics.

THE RECOVERY PHASE

The fourth phase of disaster management is the recovery phase. The recovery phase is divided into short- and long-term activities.[6] Short-term activities are defined as those that offer immediate relief and rehabilitation.[6] For the health care provider, short-term activities include vital life support and the provision of services that are necessary for patients' immediate well-being and basic comfort. Long-term activities work to restore patients' health as much as possible so they can return to the routines of daily life. This period is also known as reconstruction,[6] and during this time the patient and the health care provider must work in concert. The patient must be permitted to express concerns and needs, whereas health care providers must have the flexibility to respond and modify prior plans, if necessary, to better meet those needs.

Coping with a Different World

New Orleans evacuees who were identified as veterans needing long-term care were admitted to the Houston VA. One patient, a veteran who was admitted along with his wife (so as not to separate them), described standing in waist-deep water holding onto a tree branch for 2 days until they could be rescued. He developed open ulcers on his legs from the ordeal as a result of his diabetes, while his wife developed a urinary tract infection.

Calls from all over the United States were received from family members trying to contact relatives evacuated from New Orleans. Many patients were transferred to other VA hospitals where family members could be near. Other families, who had lost track of their sick family member, eventually located them at the Houston VA and took them home.

Two patients were unidentified. One man could not communicate because of a stroke, however eventually, another patient recognized him and he was reunited with family in California. The other patient, an elderly woman never spoke. However, after searching for her for more than 2 weeks, her family learned she had been evacuated to Houston. Her daughter phoned in hope that she had been evacuated to the Houston VA. After providing a description, the phone was held to the patient's ear. When she heard her daughter's voice, the patient exclaimed "bring me my favorite crackers to eat!"

Author's note: During the short-term phase, I had been too busy with my patients' concerns to give much thought about what I personally had experienced. Now, as my unit settled back into a more regular routine, I began to reflect on my experiences as an emergency responder.

I was particularly aware of how organization made it possible to cope with 30 new patients all at once. Had I not developed templates to aid in the processing of these new patients, I do not know how I would have coped.

My positive experience in this regard spurred me to develop a systematic process for obtaining a complete history and physical that I currently use in my own practice and use as the basis for clinical instruction of nurse practitioner students.

Indeed, I have found that my Katrina stories brought home to my students the realities of clinical practice in ways that posing hypothetical situations never could.

The long-term phase of recovery is the period of adjustment and accommodation to the realities of everyday life in the world after the disaster. This phase began after all of the evacuated patients had left the Houston VA. In the end, all but 2 of the patients were reunited with their families. These 2 men had resided in nursing homes in New Orleans that were completely destroyed and no family could be found. They both remained with the Houston VA for about 3 years until they passed away from natural causes.

Lessons Learned

After the evacuations had come to an end and the patients who had been evacuated were settled, the patient reception team met for a debriefing. Because the media were at Ellington Field even before the arrival of the patient reception team, it became obvious that security was going to be important. This had not been anticipated during preplanning meetings and, therefore, a security representative was added to the team. Another unanticipated occurrence was volunteers who started arriving at Ellington Field who did not work for the VA. Credentialing and orientation became an issue, underscoring the need to develop a method for credentialing, scheduling, and orienting volunteer staff. Issues that needed to be incorporated into future planning included the importance of technological support, such as connections for computers and phone lines, which pointed to the need for assistance with support systems at the host location.

Medical and pharmaceutical supplies were provided to cover most contingencies. However, requests for additional supplies were uncoordinated, which led to duplication of supplies that were already available. To alleviate this issue, future planning would incorporate one central requesting/approval mechanism for obtaining all appropriate supplies. Because the VA treats only adults, medical care for patients requiring pediatric or obstetric care was a challenge. Cooperative agreements with local hospitals were needed to ensure having trained staff and equipment to provide services to these populations.

During the actual disaster, command center telephone numbers were not readily available, complicating the easy establishment of communication. Preplanning to identify communication channels should be established for all key individuals. Also identified as an issue was the need to expand the volunteer base for transporters for stretchers and wheelchairs, as there were not enough personnel to manage this function.

Patients and evacuees arriving from other areas had identification and/or treatment tags in place. The additional tag added upon arrival at Ellington Field made for confusion. Therefore, the need to develop a tagging system that is plainly distinguishable from those of other entities was identified. Arrival times of the air transport or ground transport were not clearly communicated, which created confusion. An immediate intervention in the dispatch system was made to funnel this information through a single source.

Relief coverage had not been worked out. The first 24 hours were challenging until the first relief staff began to arrive; therefore, the patient reception team has been expanded to include two 12-hour shifts for the future. Finally, the patient reception team administrative structure was adjusted to account for changes needed in the future. Along with an adjusted administrative structure, the patient reception team flow chart was modified to account for all lessons learned.

SUMMARY

The patient reception team remains in existence, although its services have not been called upon since Hurricane Katrina. Drills are held, largely for ancillary personnel, with providers brought in on an as-needed basis. The team stands ready for the next challenge, knowing that the most important lesson is to expect the unexpected. Responders, who understand this and take it to heart, from the onset of the mitigation phase through to the final recovery phase, should find themselves better able to surmount the challenges they will surely face.

Author's note: I will treasure my experience as a member of the patient reception team all my life. I learned that the phases of disaster management are more than theory. I saw disaster victims experience these phases and, as their emergency care provider, I experienced them myself, albeit in different ways. I learned first-hand that a disaster leaves neither the victims nor the responders untouched.

Gradually, it began to dawn on me that while I had provided aid to the evacuees, they had given me something equally important in return—their trust. And that had made all the difference. Their faith in me inspired me to rise to unimagined challenges and in the process, further honed my skills and made me a more compassionate health care provider.

ACKNOWLEDGMENTS

Special thanks to Dian Teinert, MSN, FNP, Nurse Executive/Prime Care, Michael E. DeBakey VAMC, and Jagadeesh Kalavar, MD, Chief of Staff, Michael E. DeBakey VAMC.

REFERENCES

1. Warfield C. The disaster management cycle. 2008. Available at: http://www.gdrc. org/uem/disasters/1-dm_cycle.html. Accessed June 17, 2010.
2. Schwab AK, Eschelbach K, Brower DJ. Hazards versus disasters. In: Hazard mitigation and preparedness. New Jersey: John Wiley and Sons; 2007. p. 1–38.
3. Buchanan SA. Preservation management: emergency preparedness. In: Preservation: issues and planning. Chicago: American Library Association; 2000. p. 159–65.
4. Bush GW. The Department of Homeland Security. 2002. Available at: http://www. dhs.gov/xlibrary/assets/book.pdf. Accessed July 10, 2010.
5. National disaster medical system. Available at: http://www.hhs.gov/aspr/opeo/ ndms/index.html. Accessed July 10, 2010.
6. Perry RW, Lindell MK. Introduction to emergency planning. In: Emergency planning. New Jersey: John Wiley and Sons; 2007. p. 1–31.

Index

Note: Page numbers of article titles are in **boldface** type.

United States Postal Service

Statement of Ownership, Management, and Circulation
(All Periodicals Publications Except Requestor Publications)

1. Publication Title	2. Publication Number	3. Filing Date
Critical Care Nursing Clinics of North America	0 0 6 - 2 7 3	9/15/10

4. Issue Frequency	5. Number of Issues Published Annually	6. Annual Subscription Price
Mar, Jun, Sep, Dec	4	$130.00

7. Complete Mailing Address of Known Office of Publication (Not printer) (Street, city, county, state, and ZIP+4®)

Elsevier Inc.
360 Park Avenue South
New York, NY 10010-1710

Contact Person
Stephen Bushing

Telephone (Include area code)
215-239-3688

8. Complete Mailing Address of Headquarters or General Business Office of Publisher (Not printer)

Elsevier Inc., 360 Park Avenue South, New York, NY 10010-1710

9. Full Names and Complete Mailing Addresses of Publisher, Editor, and Managing Editor (Do not leave blank)

Publisher (Name and complete mailing address)

Kim Murphy, Elsevier, Inc., 1600 John F. Kennedy Blvd. Suite 1800, Philadelphia, PA 19103-2899

Editor (Name and complete mailing address)

Katie Hartner, Elsevier, Inc., 1600 John F. Kennedy Blvd. Suite 1800, Philadelphia, PA 19103-2899

Managing Editor (Name and complete mailing address)

Catherine Bewick, Elsevier, Inc., 1600 John F. Kennedy Blvd. Suite 1800, Philadelphia, PA 19103-2899

10. Owner (Do not leave blank. If the publication is owned by a corporation, give the name and address of the corporation immediately followed by the names and addresses of all stockholders owning or holding 1 percent or more of the total amount of stock. If not owned by a corporation, give the names and addresses of the individual owners. If owned by a partnership or other unincorporated firm, give its name and address as well as those of each individual owner. If the publication is published by a nonprofit organization, give its name and address.)

Full Name	Complete Mailing Address
Wholly owned subsidiary of	4520 East-West Highway
Reed/Elsevier, US holdings	Bethesda, MD 20814

11. Known Bondholders, Mortgagees, and Other Security Holders Owning or Holding 1 Percent or More of Total Amount of Bonds, Mortgages, or Other Securities. If none, check box. ☐ None

Full Name	Complete Mailing Address
N/A	

12. Tax Status (For completion by nonprofit organizations authorized to mail at nonprofit rates) (Check one)
The purpose, function, and nonprofit status of this organization and the exempt status for federal income tax purposes:
☐ Has Not Changed During Preceding 12 Months
☐ Has Changed During Preceding 12 Months (Publisher must submit explanation of change with this statement)

PS Form 3526, September 2007 (Page 1 of 3 (Instructions Page 3)) PSN 7530-01-000-9931 PRIVACY NOTICE: See our Privacy policy in www.usps.com

---

13. Publication Title	14. Issue Date for Circulation Data Below
Critical Care Nursing Clinics of North America	September 2010

15. Extent and Nature of Circulation			Average No. Copies Each Issue During Preceding 12 Months	No. Copies of Single Issue Published Nearest to Filing Date
a. Total Number of Copies (Net press run)			1050	1050
b. Paid Circulation (By Mail and Outside the Mail)	(1)	Mailed Outside-County Paid Subscriptions Stated on PS Form 3541. (Include paid distribution above nominal rate, advertiser's proof copies, and exchange copies)	573	523
	(2)	Mailed In-County Paid Subscriptions Stated on PS Form 3541 (Include paid distribution above nominal rate, advertiser's proof copies, and exchange copies)		
	(3)	Paid Distribution Outside the Mails Including Sales Through Dealers and Carriers, Street Vendors, Counter Sales, and Other Paid Distribution Outside USPS®	118	112
	(4)	Paid Distribution by Other Classes Mailed Through the USPS (e.g. First-Class Mail®)		
c. Total Paid Distribution (Sum of 15b (1), (2), (3), and (4))			691	635
d. Free or Nominal Rate Distribution (By Mail and Outside the Mail)	(1)	Free or Nominal Rate Outside-County Copies Included on PS Form 3541	67	63
	(2)	Free or Nominal Rate In-County Copies Included on PS Form 3541		
	(3)	Free or Nominal Rate Copies Mailed at Other Classes Through the USPS (e.g. First-Class Mail)		
	(4)	Free or Nominal Rate Distribution Outside the Mail (Carriers or other means)	67	63
e. Total Free or Nominal Rate Distribution (Sum of 15d (1), (2), (3) and (4))			67	63
f. Total Distribution (Sum of 15c and 15e)			758	698
g. Copies not Distributed (See instructions to publishers #4 (page #3))			292	352
h. Total (Sum of 15f and g)			1050	1050
i. Percent Paid (15c divided by 15f times 100)			91.16%	90.97%

16. Publication of Statement of Ownership

If the publication is a general publication, publication of this statement is required. Will be printed in the December 2010 issue of this publication. ☐ Publication not required

17. Signature and Title of Editor, Publisher, Business Manager, or Owner

Stephen R. Bushing

Stephen R. Bushing, Fulfillment/Inventory Specialist

Date September 15, 2010

I certify that all information furnished on this form is true and complete. I understand that anyone who furnishes false or misleading information on this form or who omits material or information requested on the form may be subject to criminal sanctions (including fines and imprisonment) and/or civil sanctions (including civil penalties).

PS Form 3526, September 2007 (Page 2 of 3)

Moving?

Make sure your subscription moves with you!

To notify us of your new address, find your **Clinics Account Number** (located on your mailing label above your name), and contact customer service at:

Email: **journalscustomerservice-usa@elsevier.com**

800-654-2452 (subscribers in the U.S. & Canada)
314-447-8871 (subscribers outside of the U.S. & Canada)

Fax number: **314-447-8029**

Elsevier Health Sciences Division
Subscription Customer Service
3251 Riverport Lane
Maryland Heights, MO 63043

*To ensure uninterrupted delivery of your subscription,
please notify us at least 4 weeks in advance of move.

Printed in the United States
By Bookmasters